A Stairstep Approach to Fertility

A Stairstep Approach to Fertility

Edited by Margot Edwards, R.N., M.A.

Well Women Series

The Crossing Press
Freedom, California 95019

Cover illustration and design by Betsy Bayley
Editorial assistance by Grace Darcy
Printed in the United States of America

ISBN 0-89594-3840-0 (paper)
ISBN 0-89594-385-9 (cloth)

Every effort has been made to locate copyright owners and secure permission for material used in this book.

"An Overview of Fertility" and "In Vitro Fertilization/Embryo Transfer" excerpted from *The New Our Bodies Ourselves*. © 1984 by The Boston Women's Health Collective, Inc. Reprinted by permission of Simon & Schuster, Inc.

"Fertility and Pregnancy Considerations" excerpted from *Overcoming Endometriosis* by Mary Lou Ballweg and The Endometriosis Association. © 1987 by The Endometriosis Association. Reprinted by permission of Congdon & Weed, Inc.

"Sperm Ills Cause 40% of Infertility" reprinted from *The New York Times*.

"Being in Good Health at Conception" excerpted from *Healing Yourself During Pregnancy*. © 1987 by Joy Gardner. Reprintd by permission of The Crossing Press.

"The Fasting Process" by Suza Norton excerpted from *The Holistic Health Handbook* by the Berkeley Holistic Health Center.

"Fertility Promoters" excerpted from *The Wise Woman Herbal, The Childbearing Year*. © 1989 by Susun Weed, reprinted by permission of Susun Weed.

"Non-Traditional Approaches to Infertility" by Judé d'Amato and "Learnign Through Personal Experience" by Margot Edwards, Barbara Mercer, Jessica Lipnack, and Cheryl Downing excerpted from *Mothering Magazine*. Reprinted with permission.

"Before Going to the Doctor" by Suzannah Cooper. © 1989 by Suzannah Cooper. Reprinted with permission.

"Difficulty Getting Pregnant—A Medical Problem?" excerpted from *Woman Centered Pregnancy and Birth* by Ginny Cassidy-Brinn, Francie Hornstein, and Carol Downer. © 1989 by Ginny Cassidy-Brinn, Francie Hornstein, and Carol Downer. Reprinted with permission.

"Finding the Right Doctor" excerpted from *Miracle Babies and Other Happy Endings* by Mark Perloe, M.D. and Linda Gail Christie. © 1986 by Mark Perloe, M.D. and Linda Gail Christie. Reprinted by permission of Rawson Associates, an imprint of Macmillan Publishing Company.

"New Infertility Treatment is Done in the Doctor's Office" by Charles Petit. © 1988 by The San Francisco Chronicle. Reprinted with permission.

"Donor Insemination—Traditions and Techniques" excerpted from *Having Your Baby by Donor Insemination* by Elizabeth Noble. © 1987 by Elizabeth Noble. Reprinted by permission of Houghton Mifflin Co.

"Is It Worth It? I Just Don't Know" and "He Called Me Number 27" excerpted from *Infertility: Women Speak Out*, edited by Renate Klein. © 1989 by Renate Klein. Reprinted by permission of Pandora Press.

Contents

An Explanation of the Stairstep Approach

In the wake of the excitement generated by infertility technologies, simple low cost remedies to promote conception have all but disappeared. There are safe, low-tech interventions that, in selected cases, may help regulate a menstrual cycle or increase a sperm count. If instructions for their use exist at all in written form, they are tucked away in obscure herbals or natural family planning newsletters, not described in medical journals or infertility guidebooks.

A low-tech approach to infertility is badly needed in order to promote safer ways to conceive and cut down on the exorbitant cost and emotional drain of high-tech treatment. Few would-be parents understand the impact fertility drugs have on the female body, nor are they aware that since 1979 serious questions have been raised concerning them. For example, questions raised at a seminar entitled "Ethical Issues in Human Reproduction Technology" (printed as *Birth Control and Controlling Birth and the Custom-Made Child*) and at other symposia, namely "Ethics and Eugenics: Brave New World," and "Women and Reproductive Technologies," inspired the publication, *Embryos, Ethics, and Women's Rights* in 1988.

Recently, a consumer quarterly, *Birth Journal: Issues in Perinatal Care and Education*, devoted its September 1988 issue to thorny questions about the infertility industry, calling attention to the "hucksterism" surrounding in vitro fertilization (IVF) and embryo transfer (ET). Editor Madeleine Shearer cited misplaced emphasis in developing more intricate technologies to sell to infertile couples *before* the effects and risks are ascertained in random controlled trials. "As with twilight sleep, estrogen replacement therapy, and diethylstilbestrol (DES), IVF/ET procedures are not only promoted widely within the medical community but are also actually demanded by would-be parents," even without long-term safety guarantees.

"It is understandable that women, programmed from childhood to believe that any pain is worth the opportunity to fulfill the natural role of motherhood, are willing to endure the distressing side effects of high-tech infertility treatment," commented Gena Corea in *Embryos*. "In this way of thinking," she continued, "motherhood is essential to female fulfillment, and a man must become a father if he is to be considered a mature, responsible person."

In real life, the gap between these outdated beliefs and family life as it actually exists is very wide. Nevertheless, for millions of infertile women and men, there is still the gut-wrenching grief that makes criticism of the technologies appear mean-spirited, if not downright backward.

This book brings attention to safe, low-tech alternatives that are *not* in the limelight. Admittedly, coverage is not comprehensive; this book is just a beginning. The personal accounts and reports are eye-openers for infertile people who otherwise might opt for high-tech treatment without being aware that there may be alternatives.

"For better or worse, we attempt to control things," said Barbara Eck Menning, founder of RESOLVE, an information and referral network that helps couples cope with infertility. When a woman cannot conceive, control is in short supply. As each month cancels out the long awaited and much desired pregnancy, nagging self doubt builds, compounded by disappointment and grief. The longer a woman tries and fails to become pregnant, the greater her need to do something—anything—*now*, to have a baby.

In the midst of her anguish, one way to take charge is to learn about infertility from the perspective of a health care consumer. When infertile couples know where to go and what questions to ask, they are in a much better position to make intelligent choices about infertility treatment. Medical care is a business; the patient is the buyer. To be safe and to get the best value for their health care dollars, couples have the right to know the accuracy of any proposed test and the risk of any proposed treatment. They also have the right to investigate safe, natural methods before accepting infertility technologies that are developing so rapidly that not enough time has passed to study their effects on the health of the infertile woman or man, or on the health of future generations.

Even when time is of the essence, please do not hurry into treatment before becoming informed. Take time to read this compendium. It will, in many cases, expand possibilities.

This book begins with an overview of infertility and its causes from both the female and the male perspective. Treatments for a broad spectrum of problems are also presented. Specific barriers to female conception are discussed in detail, including ectopic pregnancy, miscarriage, amenorrhea, stillbirth, sexually transmitted diseases, structural problems, endometriosis, I.U.D. and abortion infections, cervical mucus, poor health and nutrition, mechanical barriers, and genetic abnormalities.

The all-important biological clock is discussed. No matter how financially and emotionally advisable, delaying childbearing reduces the chance of conception. Over the age of thirty, one woman in four will experience difficulty conceiving. Eggs in the ovary age right along with the woman, and a history of high-dose birth control pill usage and/or I.U.D.s—coupled with a higher probability of having endometriosis—will reduce fertility even further. Women in their later reproductive years may also have had more exposure to venereal and I.U.D.-related infections that, in turn, lead to pelvic inflammatory disease (PID), a disease that permanently damages one or both of the fallopian tubes.

Despite propaganda to the contrary, male infertility problems prevent conception 35 percent to 40 percent of the time, and another 10 percent in combination with female infertility. In addition to difficulties like varicocele, mechanical blockages of the vas deferens, and sperm motility and maturation, a substantial decrease in sperm count was cited by Michael Castleman in "Toxics and Male Infertility" (*Sierra* magazine, March 1985).

This sperm drain was first discovered in 1979, when evaluations were made of healthy college students whose sperm counts were down to 20 million per milliliter as compared to 60 million in a 1974 study and 100 million in 1929. The students' semen samples were high in the toxic PCBs hexachlorobenzene and pentachlorophenol. Today, it is recognized that exposure to lead, benzene, Agent Orange, pesticides, and anesthetic gases is not only carcinogenic, but also tetragenic (contributing to birth defects), and threatening to male fertility.

Blaming Ourselves

Roughly 40 percent of all cases of infertility can be traced to the woman, 40 percent to the man, and 20 percent to the problems of both partners.

However, in a survey of infertile couples, made in 1988 by Mary Ann Draye of the University of Washington School of Nursing, 56 percent of the women believed they were the source of the problem, compared to only 19 percent of the men.

Four times as many women (49 percent) felt that their inability to conceive was a punishment for prior behavior. "They say things like, 'If only I hadn't drunk so much beer in college.'"

Although both men and women felt competent in business and other areas of their lives, infertility was a blow to self-esteem for nearly two-thirds of the women, while only 22 percent of the men were down on themselves.

This disparity points up one of the differences in the way men and women experience the crisis of infertility.

Recreational drugs like marijuana and alcohol play key roles in causing infertility in both sexes and, in the case of male marijuana use, may play a major part in the health of the baby to be born.

Prescription drugs like thalidomide and DES were recognized as reproductive hazards only *after* doing much harm. Today, DES daughters and sons (born to mothers given diethylstilbestrol, an estrogen drug mistakenly given to prevent miscarriage) are coping with the aftermath: DES-related infertility problems.

Another medical fiasco unrelated to infertility, but illustrative of the powerful side effects of exogenous hormones, was the endometrial cancer outbreak in older women who were given unopposed estrogen to reduce menopausal discomforts and stay "feminine forever."

Recently, debates about the safety of the Pill have flared up again because new and separate surveys conducted in Boston, Washington, and England say the Pill appears to be a contributing factor in the development of breast cancer.

Dr. James Schlesselman of the Uniformed Services University of the Health Sciences in Bethesda, Maryland, reviewed all medical studies made on the Pill and breast cancer after 1980. He claims that Pill use may increase breast cancer in women younger than forty-five years old ("New Studies of the Pill Suggest Link to Cancer" by Gina Kolata, *Wall Street Journal*, January 5, 1989). Admittedly, more research is needed.

After these reports appeared, The National Women's Health Network, a watchdog group in Washington, D.C., approached the Food and Drug Administration's Advisory Committee on Fertility Drugs asking them to warn prospective Pill users. According to the Network, 85 percent of all thirty-year-old American women have used the Pill, and women should be aware of its risks as well as its benefits. Today, the dangerous high-dose birth control pill, marketed as safe in the 1970s, has been replaced by a safer, low-dose counterpart. Studies of the new Pill, however, raise disquieting questions about hormone treatment and its long-term effects. (For a background on the medical administration of hormones, read *Women and the Crisis in Sex Hormones* by Barbara and Gideon Seaman and *Women's Health Care: A Guide to Alternatives* by Kay Weiss.)

We may learn from past mishaps, but there is no guarantee that hormones used today to induce ovulation in infertile women are reasonably safe over a lifetime. Hopefully, all of the currently used reproductive technologies will prove safe in twenty or thirty years (the time required for some cancers to appear), but experience shows that what is declared safe in one decade will be declared unsafe and taken off the market in another, like the high-dose Pill, DES, and unopposed estrogen replacement therapy. With history in mind, women who have difficulty conceiving can more fully understand why using a drug-free, low-tech alternative is worthy of their consideration.

Part of any natural approach to health is stress reduction. Childless couples who flinch when they bump into a pregnant woman on the street are under the greatest of pressures. In "Infertility Post-Traumatic Stress Disorder" published in the *RESOLVE National Newsletter*, April 1989, writer Ann Hill reminds us that the stress of infertility was not acknowledged until 1974, when Barbara Eck Menning explained that "infertility was the *cause* of stress, not the result of it." Hill also reported that the prestigious *New England Journal of Medicine* (December 24, 1987) finally added miscarriage to the Post-Traumatic Stress Disorder category. Hill rightfully recommended that a diagnosis of infertility be included as well.

In 1974, Menning's explanation that depressed, childless women were suffering infertility stress was badly needed to counteract the label of "psychogenic infertility." Women who could not conceive needed to be taken seriously, not called neurotic. Today, infertility is a legitimate "disease," with a battery of tests to determine every aspect. Many tests are in themselves stressful, however, and some have unwanted side effects. Today, the element of stress is sometimes given short shrift in the medical community's eagerness to get on with the infertility workup.

That stress plays a significant role in the life of a childless couple does not have to be taken as an indictment. Facing infertility *does* cause stress but, at the same time, stress can also play a role as predisposing factor. As long ago as 1978 (reported in *Mademoiselle*, March 1978), gynecologists Natalia Chapanis and John Tyson at Johns Hopkins pinned down at least part of the infertility story when they proved that stressful family relationships could trigger abnormal levels of prolactin. Excess levels of prolactin, in turn, suppress female hormones and can stop ovulation. In some cases, prolactin problems can be solved through counseling sessions alone; other cases require drugs to lower prolactin levels.

When stress is severe enough, according to Dr. John Stangel in his revised edition (1988) of *The New Fertility and Conception*, it can halt ovulation, reduce the quality and number of sperm, and "under certain very limited circumstances," interfere with the normal movements of the fallopian tubes. In *Having Your Baby By Donor Insemination: A Complete Resource Guide* (see Recommended Readings), Elizabeth Noble reported on stress associated with artificial insemination done with donor sperm in the clinic setting. Apparently, fear and embarrassment during the first try were enough to stop ovulation in the next cycle in women who otherwise ovulated regularly. Readers interested in an intelligent method of self-insemination will want to read Noble's book.

An interesting report on stress and adoption, "Is the Adoption Process an Aid to Achieving Pregnancy?" by Rose Katz et al., was published in *Social Work*, January/February 1985. The old saw that says as soon as a couple adopts a child the woman becomes pregnant was given the shaft by professionals years ago; however, there is some evidence to prove that this folklore may well be true, as shown in past research. Also, in an adoption study, it was revealed that, after applying for a child, greater numbers of younger women than usual became pregnant. Briefly, the study reported that 23.5 percent of the childless women who applied to adopt a child at Hope Cottage, a children's agency in Dallas, Texas, became pregnant as compared to the 10 percent expected to conceive. Interested social workers reviewed the literature on this phenomenon and made their own study, concluding that there was something in the process of application that freed the couples emotionally. One influence that favored pregnancy was getting the application in ahead of time, which—in the interpretation—added the missing sense of control so badly needed in a life turned upside down by infertility.

Suzannah Cooper, editor of *A Fertility Awareness and Natural Family Planning Resource Directory,* offers intelligent self-help information that includes stress reduction to childless couples willing to give it a try. While self-help may not be enough to cure a damaged fallopian tube or a blocked vas deferens, self-care is a fitting intervention for many conditions associated with infertility.

Strengthening the immune and reproductive systems, for example, is a means of regulating ovulation and improving cervical mucus and sperm health. If conception does not occur, sometimes the mind/body balance that comes from using self-help measures can prepare couples for the stressful tests and treatments that lie ahead.

One of the problems of medicalizing infertility is that self-help comes to be regarded as time-wasting foolishness. From that perspective, only the fertility specialist can help. Granted, there are conditions where the specialist's help should be sought immediately, as when a diagnostic laparoscopy is planned. In such circumstances, the patient will want a surgeon experienced in microsurgery because, if the patient is referred out by the local obstetrician, the infertility specialist will rightfully insist upon yet another laparoscopy to make a definitive diagnosis. If time is short because of age, the couple may want to go ahead with a hysterosalpingogram and semen evaluations, even as they seek out a course of self-help.

By combining low- and high-tech care in this way, the bottom line in a logical line of referral is covered—the bottom line being a person's ability to take good care of herself/himself, which is what self-help is all about.

Remember that infertility treatment is a lucrative new industry and, like any successful business, it requires promotion. The consumer (infertile couple) is subject to pep talks by health professionals and IVF clinics that raise hope to an unrealistic extent. This book provides a realistic picture of what medical treatments *and* low-tech alternatives can offer.

Just as each individual has the right to consider safe, low-tech alternatives, she also has the right to take advantage of the new reproductive technologies and make sure their effects in terms of safety and cost are clearly understood. High- and low-tech interventions *are not mutually exclusive*.

For instance, self-help to bolster health *before* having surgery can speed recovery. Herbal therapy to regulate monthly cycles and/or build healthier sperm should—if pelvic inflammatory disease (PID) is present or part of the case history—be preceded by a hysterosalpingogram to determine whether or not the fallopian tubes are damaged.

In this book, a great deal of stress is placed on the more serious female infertility problems like endometriosis (a disease that accounts for one-third of all female infertility problems) and blocked fallopian tubes (responsible for another third of female infertility problems). Women who have damaged fallopian tubes or who have tried everything in the way of treatment for endometriosis, adhesions, uterine abnormalities, antibodies to their mate's sperm, or idiopathic infertility (cause unknown) may, as a last resort, think about in vitro fertilization.

Known medically as IVF/ET (in vitro fertilization/embryo transfer), this amazing, but highly stressful, technology was originally developed for women without functioning fallopian tubes. Today, IVF/ET is offered for male as well as female problems and, increasingly, healthy fertile women consent to the rigors of IVF/ET because their husbands do not want AID (artificial insemination with donor sperm, also referred to as DI or donor insemination).

The Stairstep Approach

Instead of looking at high- and low-tech intervention as separate entities, readers are invited to consider a Stairstep Approach to solving infertility. Using the Stairstep Approach, one begins with the simpler interventions, moving into high-tech care only if necessary. If time is a factor, have medical tests done while pursuing herbal treatments or other safe alternatives.

Those who argue against this approach say it wastes valuable time; those who argue in favor of caution say it's safer, and the patient is less apt to be caught on the high-tech roller coaster that can threaten the quality of life. Let me emphasize that high-tech treatment is notoriously stressful and anxiety-producing, whereas the balancing effect of age-old treatments like acupuncture and the use of herbal remedies are relaxing to mind and body.

The Stairstep Approach also proposes that the patient function as an equal to the health care professional. Patients have the right to question their doctors, to change doctors if not satisfied, and to seek help from more than one type of professional and to secure a second opinion. In an egalitarian relationship, however, there is less room for miracles. Some couples may have to make changes on their own instead of waiting passively for the doctor to advise them. They may also have to read and do the research, instead of believing in the infallibility of every test and treatment. Whatever the outcome, they will feel better about themselves as persons.

I sincerely hope readers will consider using this Stairstep Approach to infertility conscientiously, beginning with the simpler interventions and, if necessary, slowly and with care, progressing to high-tech treatment. Unfortunately, and as I noted at the beginning of this Introduction, controlled studies of the less invasive interventions are almost nonexistent because monies are characteristically funneled into technical treatments that promise profit for the medical industries. Nevertheless, the efficacy of the simpler treatments has been proven over time, and these interventions should not be lost to this generation.

"Reproduction technology is neither a savior nor a nemesis," commented Rebecca Sarah in *Embryos*. "None of the technology . . . will save us from all of biology's inconvenience, errors, and tragedies.

"Nor can it guarantee healthy babies, or pregnancy when and only when we want it. There are reasons why we have come to expect perfection and why doctors think they can provide that perfection. I think it is this very expectation that leads to the misuse of technology and, as a result, to most of the problems associated with it."

Margot Edwards, R.N., M.A.

SECTION I

An Overview of Fertility

Many of us have childbearing problems which cause us difficulty and emotional pain. After years of using birth control and being voluntarily childless, we are confronted with the reality that when we consciously decide to have children, we are unable to conceive or unable to carry a pregnancy to term.

We can learn to deal with potential problems and actual crises in two ways. First, we will want to have a general awareness that things may go wrong. We can tuck away such information to be used sometime in the future, if necessary. The knowledge itself can't hurt us, but if it upsets us, we can hold dialogues with ourselves, our partners, or our friends. Second, if we do suspect we can't conceive, if we miscarry or have other problems, we will want more specific information to answer our questions: What is happening? What shall I do? Where shall I get help? How shall I cope? What is my next step? What other questions shall I ask?

We and our doctors are practicing sound preventive medicine when we ask our questions as strongly as we can, and they answer them respectfully and to the best of their knowledge.

We can also seek out the physiological causes of our problems by reading all the available literature, learning about diagnostic procedures and available treatments, asking for test results, and insisting on further tests if we are not satisfied. We can develop emotional strengths to cope with what we are living through. Crises may produce feelings of isolation, fear, anger, grief, guilt, and helplessness, as well as obsessions and fantasies. During such times, we need sympathetic support from our partners, our friends, and others who have had similar experiences. We need to be able to reach out to others.

Infertility

Infertility is defined by most doctors as the inability to conceive after a year or more of sexual relations without contraception. The category includes women who conceive but can't maintain a pregnancy long enough for the fetus to become viable (able to live outside the mother). You have the right to consider yourself infertile whenever you begin to feel concerned about your failure to become pregnant. Infertility may be a temporary or permanent state, depending on your problem and on the available treatments. Many people are surprised to learn that infertility is fairly common. *Between 15 and 20 percent* of couples *in the United States are infertile.* In 35 percent of these cases, male factors are responsible; in 35 percent, female factors are responsible; in 30 percent, combined factors are responsible.

Infertility appears to be on the rise. It now affects over ten million people. Some major factors which have led to this increase are the rise in STD-caused infections, which may lead to permanent damage to the reproductive system, widespread use of the Pill, which causes ovulatory problems; the I.U.D., which contributes to infertility by causing PID (pelvic inflammatory disease) after insertion; women's decision to delay childbearing into their thirties, when fertility decreases slightly and the increase in environmental and industrial toxic products, which can affect both men's and women's reproductive systems. A badly done abortion, or one which has not been properly followed up, can cause infections which, if not treated, affect fertility.

Though up until now one myth has held that infertility is the woman's problem, it has become clear that the man and woman must be diagnosed and treated together. If the man has the problem, then treatment of the woman alone has no value and usually involves many needless, painful, and expensive tests. A man, because of his anatomy, is easier to diagnose, and semen analysis is one of the logical tests to perform first.

Another myth is that infertility is not treatable. *In fact, 50 percent of infertile people treated are able to achieve a pregnancy!*

When you seek help for infertility, it is crucial to have a good relationship with your doctor. Find someone who specializes in infertility. The best infertility specialists are reproductive endocrinologists, who are obstetrician-gynecologists with two additional years of training in the field of infertility. If you don't have confidence in your doctor's methods, go elsewhere. Get a second opinion; that is your right.

It's important that your doctor be respectful of your body, mind, and feelings; aware of your pain and strong emotions, and available to you when you need him or her. It's the responsibility of your nurse and doctor to explain words and procedures so that you can fully understand—it may take you awhile, because you are learning a new language and may be under stress. It is often helpful to make a written list of questions to take with you to each appointment, and bring your partner or a friend with you.

You may need help from your partner, close friends, or an infertility support group to obtain the necessary tests and diagnostic procedures you have learned about. Become as familiar with your own body's functions as you can.

Emotional Responses to Infertility

Infertility is a life crisis. It is usually unexpected; often we don't know how to cope with the feelings raised by the experience of discovering we are infertile. There is an initial reaction of shock and denial.

Often, it seems as if your life is on hold, as you postpone changing jobs, going back to school, etc., because "six months from now you will be pregnant."

When women you know have children, it may be hard for you to relate to them. Feelings of envy, jealousy, and "why them and not me" are common. Because holidays are so child-centered, they can become stressful, lonely, and depressing times for you. You may feel isolated from your friends and your mate. You may each react differently to the infertility crisis.

Anger is a common feeling, but it is hard to know where and toward whom to direct it. We tend to look for a reason for our infertility. We may feel that something we did in the past caused our present inability to conceive. Some people irrationally think that past abortions (even though properly performed), masturbation, unusual sex practices, etc., have caused this form of "punishment." They do not cause infertility, but our minds can trick us into believing it and make us feel terribly guilty. Depression, sadness, and despair are common.

Causes of Infertility

Infertility is based on several physiological events and their timing. Your partner must produce sperm of sufficient quantity, quality, and motility (ability to swim). You must produce a healthy ovum. Sperm must be deposited in your vagina and move upward through cervical mucus to meet the ovum while it is still in the tube. (Timing of sexual relations is important, since an ovum may live as little as twelve or twenty-four hours, a sperm as little as one or two days.) Once the sperm and ovum have united, the resulting group of cells must implant properly in the uterine lining and proceed to grow. The usual order of tests done in an infertility checkup is based on an organized attempt to check all the links in this chain of events.

A man may be infertile because of:

1. Problems of production and maturation of the sperm. These can be caused by previous infection, especially after puberty, such as mumps; undescended testicles; chemical and environmental factors; drugs, and occupational hazards. Taking hot saunas and baths can cause overly high temperatures in the scrotal sac, an effect which lasts a few months. In addition, a varicocele (a varicose vein in the scrotum) can affect sperm production.

2. Problems with the movement (motility) of the sperm. These may be due to chronic prostatitis and abnormally low or very thick semen. In addition, certain drugs used to treat emotional disorders can affect sperm motility.

3. Problems of conduction. These can result from scar tissue in the delicate passageways through which the sperm travel; this may be caused by infections or untreated STD. (Intentional blockage is accomplished by vasectomy.)

4. Inability to deposit the sperm into the cervix. This can be caused by sexual dysfunction, such as impotence or premature ejaculation, as well as by structural problems in the penis; for example, when the opening is either on the top or underside of the penis instead of at the tip. Spinal cord injuries and various neurological diseases can also contribute to this problem.

5. Other factors affecting male fertility. These include poor nutrition

and poor general health. Researchers recommend that men eat well and increase their intake of zinc, vitamin C, and vitamin E.

A woman may be infertile because of:

1. Mechanical barriers which prevent the union of the sperm and ovum, caused by scarring on the tubes or ovaries from previous PID or from certain I.U.D.s (particularly the Dalkon Shield). There is a 9 percent higher risk of developing PID if a woman is using an I.U.D., and this risk is increased sixfold if she has a Dalkon Shield. Untreated STD, such as gonorrhea, can also cause scarring and tubal blockage.

2. Endometriosis can cause scarring and tubal blockage.

3. Endocrine problems. Failure to ovulate regularly or irregular menstrual periods may be due to a malfunction of the ovaries, pituitary, hypothalamus, thyroid, or adrenal glands. Normally, several specific hormones are secreted at specific times in the menstrual cycle. If any one of these is not produced, or produced in insufficient quantity, the whole cycle can be thrown off. In addition, when ovulation is unpredictable, the chances of conception are decreased, as women cannot count on a consistent cycle with a known fertile time. Women often develop amenorrhea (absence of menstrual periods) following the use of birth control pills, which can result in infertility. Women who have irregular periods or who are older when they start their first menstrual periods seem to be more prone to this so-called "post-Pill syndrome."

4. Structural problems in the uterus or cervix due to congenital problems or DES exposure *in utero* can cause infertility by preventing conception or affecting the normal growth and expansion of the uterus during pregnancy. If the cervix is affected, miscarriage may result.

5. Cervical mucus of an incorrect consistency or pH (an expression of acidity and alkalinity) can act as a barrier to the normal movement of the sperm up into the vagina.

6. Other factors, such as genetic abnormalities, extreme weight loss or weight gain, excessive exercise, poor nutrition, and environmental and industrial toxins, may affect a woman's fertility. Infections, such as those caused by T-mycoplasma and chlamydia, can cause infertility by changing the quality of cervical mucus and possibly causing early miscarriage.

Infertility also takes the form of repeated miscarriage or stillbirths. In these instances, conception is not the problem; there is an inability to carry a pregnancy to live birth.

A couple may have a combination of problems which results in infertility. Some shared causes are: 1. *Immunological response*. You or your partner may have sperm antibodies which tend to destroy the sperm's action by immobilizing them or causing them to clump. 2. *Simple lack of knowledge*. Neither of you may know when you are fertile, how often to have intercourse during this time, or what to do during intercourse to make pregnancy more possible.

Finally, for 10 percent of infertile couples, physicians cannot specifically diagnose any cause for their infertility ("normal infertility"). These couples are told everything is "normal," and they can do nothing but wait. This finding can be one of the hardest to cope with—the idea that there is nothing that can be done. You may be told that your problems are all in your head. This kind of attitude is not helpful at all. Often you may be victims of a condition whose cause or cure has yet to be discovered. We must all press for more research.

Masters and Johnson stated that one out of five couples who attended their infertility clinic over a twenty-four-year period conceived within three months with no treatment other than use of this basic information: if your menstrual cycle is regular, whether it be long or short, you will probably ovulate fourteen days (give or take twenty-four hours either way) before the beginning of your next period. In other words, you should try to become pregnant on the thirteenth, fourteenth, and fifteenth days before your next period. During these three days, spacing your lovemaking is important. A man's sperm production decreases if he makes love too often, so you should have intercourse no more than once every thirty or thirty-six hours to keep active sperm in your genital tract during that period of time. It is wise to have intercourse two days before this three-day period to stimulate your partner's sperm production.

If your uterus is not tilted back, the most effective position for intercourse will be with your partner above and facing you, and a folded pillow under your hips to raise them. (If your uterus is tilted back, use three or four pillows.) Use no artificial lubricant, such as jellies or creams, and never douche afterward. If lubrication is necessary, saliva is the safest choice. He should penetrate as deeply as possible, and when he reaches orgasm, he should stop thrusting and hold quite still, deep in your vagina.

Approximately 60 to 70 percent of the sperm are contained in the first part of the ejaculate. Since it usually takes about twenty minutes for sperm to travel through the cervical mucus up to the uterus and fallopian tubes, it is a good idea to stay on your back with your knees elevated for about thirty minutes. (Some women recommend douching with baking soda thirty minutes before intercourse to change the consistency of cervical mucus and make it less viscous, so that sperm encounter less resistance.)

Though these methods may at times seem too mechanical and may make you tense, try to keep in your minds and hearts your good feelings for each other.

If your menstrual cycle is very irregular, determine the time you ovulate by using a basal temperature chart, monitoring the type and amount of your cervical mucus, and asking a fertility awareness group or your doctor for more help if you need it.

Many couples know that infertility and planned sex really affect their sexual life. Spontaneity in lovemaking decreases. You have to plan your sex life around your menstrual cycle; it becomes less an act of loving and pleasure and more a medically necessary response. Recording the time of your sexual relations on a temperature chart may make you feel like nothing is private or sacred in your life anymore!

You can determine from the chart if you are ovulating or not and can time your sex to coincide. If you are ovulating normally, from the time of your last period until ovulation you'll have a fluctuating, low temperature (around 98 degrees or less). About the time of ovulation, there's usually a sharp dip followed by a rise of half a degree or more. Some cycles show just a rise with no preceding dip. The higher plateau (usually around 98.4 degrees) is maintained until the day before your next period, when it drops again. Your doctor will give you a chart, or you can get one from your nearest Planned Parenthood Association.

You must wait at least two cycles to begin to interpret the chart with any degree of accuracy.

Other Causes of Infertility

PMS/Hypothyroidism

Women with pre-menstrual syndrome (PMS) who are also infertile may find that thyroid therapy resolves the problem. An easy way to discover low thyroid activity (hypothyroidism) is to place a thermometer on the night table before retiring. Immediately upon waking, and with a mimimum of movement, place the thermometer under the arm and allow it to stay there for five to ten minutes. If body temperature is lower than 98.6 degrees it might be wise to contact a physician and arrange for a thyroid test.

Cigarettes

Cigarettes not only affect fertility but also lower the birth weights of smokers' children.

A recent survey of pregnant women found that smokers were 72 percent as fertile as nonsmokers in a typical month. In the first month of trying to conceive, 38 percent of nonsmokers became pregnant; only 28 percent of the smokers conceived. After six months of trying to conceive, the study said, 90 percent of the nonsmokers succeeded as opposed to only 76 percent of the smokers.

Marijuana

Long-term marijuana use can seriously affect the reproductive systems of women and men. Long-term use is defined as having at least one "joint" a day (or seven a week).

In females, marijuana reduces the size of the uterus and ovaries. Hormone output is lessened, resulting in the disruption of ovulation and leading either to abnormal menstruation or its complete cessation. Statistics indicate that women users are three times more likely to have irregular menstrual periods than non-users.

In males, marijuana reduces the number of sperm cells and their motility. Researchers noted an increase in the number of abnormal sperm cells with large quantities of damaged chromosomes. The seminal vesicle and prostate gland shrink, resulting in a reduction in testosterone output.

Diagnosis

A complete infertility workup with all the diagnostic tests can take four or five menstrual cycles. Many of the tests have to be scheduled at specific times in your cycle and can't be combined. An infertility workup is expensive, and, unfortunately, medical insurance coverage in most cases is poor. The tests for women are invasive, painful, often undignified, and emotionally exhausting.

Though the sequence of diagnostic studies will vary both with doctors and individuals, it will include some or all of the following:

1. *A general physical and medical history of both man and woman.*
2. *A pelvic examination of the woman.* Your reproductive tract, breasts, and general development will be checked. You will want to tell your doctor about your menstrual history, including the onset and pattern of your menstrual periods; about any previous pregnancies, episodes of STD, or abortions; about your use of birth control; about your sexual relations (frequency, position, and related feelings); about where you live and what your job is, for environmental toxins may have affected you.
3. *A basal temperature chart.* You will take your temperature daily with a special thermometer and record it on the chart given to you.
4. *Semen analysis.* Your partner will ejaculate a sample of semen into a clean container. It must be kept at body temperature and examined as soon as possible under a microscope to determine the sperm count and motility. A count over twenty million sperm per cubic centimeter is considered in the normal range; below ten million per cubic centimeter is considered poor. Yet men with low sperm counts *can* impregnate. The sperm must be able to swim in a forward motion and at least 60 percent should be normal in size and shape.

Repeat the semen analysis at least one more time, since a man's sperm can fluctuate in count and motility for many reasons. If the semen analysis is abnormal, your partner should pursue his own diagnosis before you have further tests done. Any diagnosis of infertility can make things difficult for both man and woman.

If all male factors are normal, study of the woman will continue. You may need to have a

5. *Post-coital test (Sims-Hühner test).* Just before you expect to ovulate, you will make love with your partner and within several hours will arrive at your doctor's office without washing or douching. The doctor will take a small amount of mucus from your vagina and cervix to be studied for the number of live, active sperm. A normal test result shows that sperm have the ability to penetrate cervical mucus and live in this environment. This test may be combined with another, also done at this time in your cycle, called

6. *Tubal insufflation (Rubin test).* A gas, carbon dioxide, is blown under carefully monitored pressure into your uterus through the cervix. Normally, it will escape out the tubes into the surrounding cavity, causing shoulder pain when you sit up. (It is eventually absorbed into your body.) If the gas doesn't pass readily, pressure will be increased within safe limits. If the results are abnormal, it may be repeated or confirmed by X-ray studies. The Rubin test indicates that blockages exist but can't tell where they are located. As a result, this test is now often being replaced by the

7. *Utero-tubogram*, also called *hysterosalpingogram*, which allows for direct visualization of the tubes and provides a permanent record that can be used for comparison if future X-rays are needed. Doctors usually perform this procedure in the first part of the cycle, before ovulation, to prevent possible X-ray exposure of a fertilized egg if conception has occurred. (Whenever you have X-rays, you are irradiating all future eggs.) It involves injecting a harmless dye into the vagina and uterus. The dye should pass up through the uterus to the tubes and out into the abdominal cavity. A series of X-rays are taken during this process. The dye then passes out into the surrounding cavity and your body reabsorbs it. This test can be painful, especially if pressure is used to get the dye to pass through the tubes. Practitioners may give you local cervical anesthesia or an oral medication to help you relax before this test.

8. *Blood levels of the hormones* estrogen, progesterone, and prolactin, as well as urine tests, will be done to determine if your hormone levels are normal and whether ovulation has occurred.

9. *An endometrial biopsy* is another test to determine whether you are ovulating. It can be done any time from a week after ovulation is suspected

to the first day of your period. The doctor inserts a small instrument into your uterus after partially dilating your cervix (this will cause some unpleasant cramping), scrapes a tiny piece of tissue from the lining of the uterus (endometrium), and sends it to be examined microscopically. Tissue formed while progesterone is being produced (after ovulation) is different from tissue formed under the influence of estrogen (before ovulation) or in the absence of hormonal influence. Hormonal levels in urine and blood serum can also be helpful in diagnosis of ovulation and the total hormone picture. If s/he finds no problem, your doctor may want to do a *culdoscopy* or *laparoscopy*—hospital procedures which allow direct visualization of the tubes, ovaries, exterior of the uterus, and the surrounding cavities. In culdoscopy, a small incision is made in the back wall of your vagina; in laparoscopy, an incision is made near your navel. Both tests are done under general or spinal anesthesia and can yield a great deal of information.

When you are going through these tests, once again your sex life comes under "scientific scrutiny."

You also become a "public" figure. Relatives ask you, "Well, has it happened yet?" Or, worse, they don't say anything, but they look at you and sigh a lot. People you hardly know may comment on your problem. Hopefully, during these times, you can support each other and learn to keep both your sense of humor and your sense of the awesomeness and privacy of sexuality.

Treatment

In 90 percent of cases, a reason is found for the infertility. Your doctor should talk with you both and outline a plan for treatment.

In general, male problems respond poorly to medical treatment. However, various hormones, also used to treat female infertility (clomiphene citrate, HCG [human chorionic gonadotropin], and HMG [human menopausal gonadotropin]), are now being tried with good success in the male. A varicocele can be corrected surgically, with a rise in sperm count and motility usually seen three months after surgery. The stress of waiting to hear the results can take its toll on couples. Insemination with your mate's sperm is sometimes used if the count is low, in the hope that, with proper placement at the time of insemination, chances of conception will be increased. If infection is causing a decrease in sperm motility, it may be corrected by treatment with antibiotics.

For women, treatment for endocrine disorders currently offers the highest degree of success. Doctors use a variety of drugs to correct hormonal imbalances, to help induce ovulation, and to correct problems in the luteal phase (after ovulation). The main drugs used to induce ovulation are clomiphene citrate; HCG, a hormone extracted from the human placenta; and HMG (trade name Pergonal), extracted from the urine of menopausal women.

Clomiphene citrate was introduced in the 1960s and is a commonly used infertility drug. It is taken orally on the fifth to the tenth day of the cycle. It appears to act directly upon the hypothalamus in the brain and causes it to produce more of the hormones FSH (follicle-stimulating hormone) and LH (luteinizing hormone), which then stimulate the ovary to ripen and release an egg. About 80 percent of women will ovulate with the help of this drug, and about 50 percent will become pregnant, with a 5 to 10 percent incidence of multiple births. Some women experience breast tenderness, hot flashes, headaches, blurred vision, and throbbing feelings in the ovaries at the time of ovulation while on clomiphene citrate. A potential complication is hyperstimulation of the ovary which, if undetected, may result in ovarian damage. Ideally, women on this medication should have a checkup at the end of each cycle to be sure this complication isn't developing.

HCG is often combined with clomiphene citrate and given intramuscularly near the time of expected ovulation. It acts like LH on the ovary and helps the developing egg ripen and release.

HMG, a very potent hormone used to induce ovulation, should only be prescribed by an infertility specialist. Treatment with HMG involves frequent injections of the drug and often daily visits to a laboratory where blood and urine are examined for estrogen levels. Some doctors also use ultrasound to monitor the development of the ovarian follicle(s). By monitoring these levels carefully, the danger of multiple eggs being released from the ovary and consequent multiple births is reduced. Ovarian hyperstimulation is also a possible complication of use of this drug.

Bromocriptine is another drug used to treat female infertility due to high levels of the hormone prolactin in the blood. In breastfeeding mothers, prolactin levels are normally elevated. Occasionally this hormone is elevated in the infertile woman as well. It appears that high prolactin levels can disturb normal ovulatory patterns. In such cases, bromocriptine is taken orally until prolactin levels fall and normal ovulation results.

Problems in the luteal phase of the cycle may be treated with any or all of the following: clomiphene citrate, HCG, and natural progesterone. Natural progesterone is available in vaginal suppositories or given via intramuscular injections. You usually insert the suppositories twice daily, starting after ovulation. Synthetic forms of progesterone are not advised, as they can be harmful to fetal development in an unsuspected pregnancy.

Surgical techniques can often correct cervical weakness and various structural problems of the uterus. Microsurgery is a special type of surgery used to repair tubes and to remove adhesions. Laser surgery using the carbon dioxide laser is also being used, often in combination with microsurgery, to remove scar tissue or endometrial adhesions. Endometriosis can be treated surgically and/or with oral medications. Cervical mucus problems, depending on their cause, are treated with hormones or a form of steroid (not a common treatment; effects are fluid retention and masking of other infections). Special douches can help if the mucus is overly acid.

Women often have a combination of problems, and their treatment may involve a combination of several medications, many of which are expensive. It is important to understand how these drugs work, how they affect you, and how long you should use them.

Shared infertility problems are usually treated by separate doctors. The man goes to a urologist and the woman to a gynecologist or infertility specialist. *Your doctors must communicate with each other.* For any couple with a shared problem, the potential to achieve pregnancy is improved dramatically if even one member of the couple can be treated and helped. If both of you can be helped, then your chances are excellent.

In all cases, there is a 5 percent spontaneous cure rate (a cure without any treatment whatever). Often, after many years of trying, pregnancy will finally occur. We do not understand these spontaneous cures, but the fact that they do happen is a source of hope when all else fails.

In "inconclusive" fertility there are usually no clear-cut medical reasons. It can be difficult for you and your doctor to know when to stop the tests, to put away the thermometer, or to stop various treatments. Your feelings of hopefulness may give way to depression, often a painful process. In the case of "conclusive" or "absolute" infertility, you have the facts from the doctor. You must now adjust to that reality and re-examine your life. You may feel as if "the death of all your babies" has occurred. You may feel grief for the loss of a part of womanhood or manhood, for the parts of you that don't work or have been cut out of you. If you deny or repress this feeling of grief, you prolong the process of its resolution. Somewhere inside, you are dealing with the experience. You have the choice of living it as consciously and directly as you can or suppressing these very natural but painful emotions. Sometimes the pain of infertility is never completely resolved but is accepted as a familiar ache, which may recur, unpredictably, throughout life. Grieving often takes a long time. To do your "grief work," the support of friends, family, and other people who have experienced infertility, can be helpful.

From *The New Our Bodies Ourselves*

SECTION 2

Female Infertility

Introduction

At the beginning of Section 1, infertility was defined as the inability to conceive after at least a year of sexual intercourse without contraception. Often, however, women *do* conceive, are filled with the joy of anticipation, only to lose the child-to-be through spontaneous abortion (miscarriage), or ectopic pregnancy (where the egg starts to grow in the fallopian tube instead of the uterus).

In this section, we explore these causes of female infertility, as well as amenorrhea and endometriosis. Mary Lou Ballweg and The Endometriosis Association discuss aspects of endometriosis in their excellent article, "Fertility and Pregnancy Considerations," and we include a brief overview of of sexually transmitted disease (STD) and its effect on women who desire to become pregnant.

Miscarriage

One miscarriage does not mean you are infertile. There is a 70 per cent chance that you will have a successful pregnancy even after two miscarriages. However, if you have two or more in a row, you may want to begin investigating. Plan with your doctor to check out each detail of your next pregnancy as it progresses, including possible reasons for any spotting or cramps, definite ways to deal with contingencies, tests to be made as they become necessary, and so forth. You will need encouragement in this project from your partner, friends, and/or a support group, possibly one geared to childbearing problems.

The time following a miscarriage is difficult. Physically, your body may still feel pregnant for a while, your breasts full and tender, your stomach enlarged. You may continue spotting for several weeks. If you have increased flow or odd- or foul- smelling discharge or a fever, contact your doctor. It is usually safe to have sexual intercourse after four to six weeks when your cervix is closed and there is less risk of infection.

You may not believe what is happening. During the miscarriage, feelings of helplessness may develop as cramping and bleeding increase. Many women fear that they may bleed to death. Having to go to the hospital may intensify your anxiety and fear.

You will almost always feel grief and anger. You will need family and friends. Feelings of grief are often complicated by guilt, which can cause tension between you and your partner. You may wonder if either of you did something "wrong" (too much activity, too much sex, not enough good food, etc.). You will be blaming each other unnecessarily, for such factors rarely cause miscarriage. Dispelling the tension will take awhile, longer for some than for others. It is best if you acknowledge and talk out your feelings. The effects of the miscarriage can last for months. On the date when the baby would have been born, there is usually a resurgence of grief.

If you experience more than three miscarriages, it is important to see a doctor who specializes in this problem. You will need one who is skilled and also compassionate and understanding of the losses you have experienced, and of how very precious these pregnancies were to you. Such doctors are rare. Your helplessness and hopelessness may increase if you begin (or return to) treatments for your infertility and start working on becoming pregnant again.

> *A woman who has had three miscarriage in a row is considered a "habitual aborter" by doctors. At this point, the usual treatment is hormones. According to an item in the British Medical Journal, researchers followed twenty-one "habitual aborters" who were not given any active treatment to prevent miscarriage. Only one woman in the study failed to achieve a live birth, and 75 percent delivered normal, healthy infants. Researchers recommend that— except in extreme cases—women who have recurrent spontaneous abortions should not be treated medically; rather, they should be encouraged to continue trying to have babies.*

Ectopic Pregnancy

Ectopic pregnancy is another form of infertility. Pregnancy loss results because the fertilized egg starts developing in the tube instead of in the uterus. Between 5 and 10 percent of women who have had previous tubal surgery may experience ectopic pregnancy, but it can happen to any woman. Ectopic pregnancies are on the rise because of the increased incidence of pelvic inflammatory disease (PID) and use of IUDs, which can result in scar formation on the tubes or inflammation of the uterine lining, which then "resists" implantation of the fertilized egg. If you're old enough to bear a child, have had intercourse, and feel abdominal pains you don't understand, it's possible you have an ectopic pregnancy.

Because all the hormonal changes are similar to those of a normal early pregnancy, you can have all the early signs of pregnancy (fatigue, nausea, missed period, and breast tenderness). As the pregnancy progresses, causing pressure in the tube, symptoms such as stabbing pain, cramps, or a dull ache may become severe. In addition, you may or may not have menstrual-type bleeding. Ectopic pregnancy is sometimes misdiagnosed as an early spontaneous abortion. It is essential that any tissue passed from the uterus be checked for developing fetal tissue, that an ultrasound be done, and/or that a beta subunit blood test be done as well. This test can pick up levels of HCG in the blood. If levels are low, an ectopic pregnancy should be suspected. *Ectopic pregnancy requires immediate treatment.* There is danger of severe blood loss and shock if the tube ruptures.

If the doctor detects an ectopic pregnancy early enough, s/he may be able to remove the pregnancy and save the tube. In some cases, it is necessary to remove the whole tube and/or the adjacent ovary. Careful surgical technique is important; the less bleeding and consequent adhesions and scar tissue, the better the chance for a normal pregnancy later. In any case, if you have already had a tubal pregnancy there is a higher risk of having another.

You may have all the feelings that result from a miscarriage. In addition, you may have had internal bleeding, and you will have had the trauma of an emergency surgical operation. The outlook for future pregnancies is somewhat changed by this experience: you may feel depressed and frightened by the possibility that this could happen again.

From *The New Our Bodies Ourselves*

Amenorrhea

Amenorrhea is defined as the abnormal absence or suppression of the menstrual discharge and is divided into categories: (1) primary amenorrhea—when a woman has not had a menstrual period by the time menarche usually begins (eighteen years); (2) secondary amenorrhea—cessation of menstruation after at least one period.

Although there are many natural causes for amenorrhea— including pregnancy, menopause, breastfeeding, and congenital defects—there are also outside causes. These include cysts or tumors, heavy athletic activity, too little body fat, dieting, prior use of the Pill, some drugs, hormonal imbalance, starvation, chromosome abnormalities, disease, anemia, emotional problems, and stress.

Our national preoccupation with dieting and physical exercise can result in amenorrhea for some women. When dieting, women must be sure their weight loss does not exceed 10 to 15 percent below their minimum weight. Excessive exercise also causes amenorrhea.

Because it often causes infertility, doctors tend to pay more attention to amenorrhea than they do to painful menstruation or pre-menstrual syndrome.

Treatment

For unusually light periods or for amenorrhea, a woman might try pennyroyal leaf tea (please do not use pennyroyal oil; it may be toxic) brewed at one teaspoon per cup of water. If body weight has fallen to 10 or 15 percent below normal weight, putting on some weight may solve the problem.

Severe anemia (a reduction in hemoglobin or in the volume of packed red blood cells) can also cause amenorrhea. Anemia itself is a complex illness and occurs four times as often in women as in men. Iron-deficiency anemia is the most common form of anemia in women and is best prevented through an iron-rich diet including iron supplements such as ferrous gluconate or chelated iron.

If amenorrhea occurs while a woman is taking the Pill, vitamin B6, folic acid, and vitamin E supplements may help.

In their excellent book, *Women and the Crisis in Sex Hormones*, Barbara and Gideon Seaman suggest that, instead of using drugs or hormones, women with amenorrhea try a high-protein diet and include supplements. They, too, suggest vitamins B6 and E, and folic acid, but also include the vitamin C complex, zinc, and add selenium to the vitamin E.

The Seamans suggest that underweight women with amenorrhea follow a higher calorie diet that includes wheat germ oil and vitamin E.

Post-Pill amenorrhea (when menstruation does not return after the woman stops taking the Pill) occurs most frequently in women whose periods were irregular even before they took the Pill. Studies indicate that starting to menstruate late and using the Pill early are predisposing factors for post-Pill amenorrhea. Sadly, these studies also reveal that the risks of long-term, possibly permanent, infertility are highest in women who did not have a child before taking the Pill.

Despite these studies and their unhappy findings, most post-Pill amenorrhea problems will spontaneously correct themselves within two years and, in some cases, in just a few months. Barbara and Gideon Seaman believe that, with good nutrition and proper supplements, correction can take place more quickly.

According to the Seamans, "Some fertility treatments, aside from . . . nutritional regimens . . . are so dangerous in themselves that no woman should agree to them just to get her periods back. If she cannot bear the anxiety, her doctor may suggest Provera after three months, and low doses of Clomid after six.

Endometriosis

Endometriosis is a disease that occurs when some of the tissue that usually lines the uterus (endometrium) grows in other parts of the body. This growth, often referred to as nodules, tumors, lesions, or growths, most often occurs in the pelvic area where it spreads to the ovaries, ligaments, fallopian tubes, the outside surface of the uterus, and the bowel. It can also spread to the bladder, intestines, or even to distant parts of the body, including the arm, lung, or even the head.

These displaced growths build up and respond to the hormonal influences of the woman's cycle by bleeding during the menstrual period. Because it can find no way to leave the body as the menstrual flow does, the buildup may cause inflammation, internal bleeding, and it may cause cysts and scar tissue.

Mistakenly called "the career woman's disease," endometriosis affects an estimated 15 percent of American women in all walks of life, some with children. Half become infertile, although only a small portion of women with endometriosis experience scarring of the fallopian tubes. Why endometriosis causes infertility in the absence of scarring cannot be explained.

Endometriosis is associated with one-third of all female infertility cases. In women without symptoms, it is sometimes diagnosed by laparotomy of laparoscopy.

Although doctors sometimes diagnose endometriosis by palpation (an external examination by the hands) or by pelvic examination, a definitive diagnosis is made by a laparoscopic examination. Curiously enough, some women with widespread endometriosis suffer little pain, while others with minimal endometriosis experience severe pain. One explanation for this is that the inflammation associated with any fresh implants triggers prostaglandin (a substance involved in pain physiology) secretion, whereas older endometrial lesions no longer have this effect. To add to the confusion, one-third of all women with endometriosis are without symptoms.

There is no known cure for endometriosis, nor is the disease process understood. Years of menstruation uninterrupted by pregnancy appears to favor onset. Less known is a suspicious link with the high-dose birth control pill. According to the Endometriosis Association newsletter (Volume 8, Number 5), studies done by a distinguished group of research centers revealed a link between endometriosis and high-dose oral contraceptive use. Although more research is needed before conclusions are final, these studies found that women using oral contraceptives were at greater risk for endometriosis.

Ironically, medical treatment prescribed the Pill to "dry up" endometriosis lesions by suppressing menstrual bleeding in order to provide relief—

hopefully—from monthly pain; however, danazol (a derivative of the male hormone testosterone) is the preferred treatment today. Danazol is marketed in the United States as Danocrine and, in Canada, as Cyclomen.

Although danazol has unfortunate masculinizing effects, women take it for unrelenting pain and/or to shrink endometriosis implants enough to become pregnant. Surgical treatment includes a wide range of options including scraping, cutting, or cauterizing the implants, excision of the implants via laparoscopy, laparotomy (abdominal surgery) or laser surgery, or hysterectomy (which does not always eliminate pain). Unfortunately, the surgery itself sometimes causes more scarring (adhesions).

Dr. David Redwine, a specialist in the treatment of endometriosis, has overturned many of the traditional beliefs about this disease. He believes endometriosis is congenital. It is found largely on the peritoneum (the lining of the abdominal cavity and the inner organs) and, when excised, there is a low rate of recurrence. Pain that returns is not usually caused by new lesions, but by existent implants missed by the surgeon. Redwine himself claims a recurrence rate of less than 10 percent, crediting a "near contact" technique that helps him detect endometrial lesions. Implants, he says, are not only black as they usually are described, but can also be clear as well as white, blue, yellow, and red.

Surgical excision provides tissue for biopsy, and Dr. Redwine bases many of his concepts upon extensive research with the tissue. For information, write to Nancy Peterson, R. N., at St. Charles Medical Center, 2500 NE Neff Rd., Bend, OR 97701.

Women with endometriosis will find their best resource is the Endometriosis Association founded by Mary Lou Ballweg in 1980. This Advocacy group maintains a registry with thousands of case histories at the University of Washington and publishes an informative and supportive newsletter. In 1988, Ballweg and the Association compiled a book entitled, *Overcoming Endometriosis: New Help from the Endometriosis Association*, from which the following article "Fertility and Pregnancy Considerations" is taken.

By *Margot Edwards; R.N., M.A.*

Fertility and Pregnancy Considerations

About 30 to 40 percent of women with endometriosis are infertile, and endometriosis is the cause of infertility in about 30 percent of all infertile women, according to infertility specialists. For women with endometriosis, infertility is more likely to result as the disease progresses, with less infertility in the early stages.

The reasons for infertility in endometriosis are not known. A number of factors probably contribute: damage to the ovaries and fallopian tubes by the disease; adhesions and scar tissue on these and other organs due to the disease and sometimes due to surgery; irregular periods; painful sex resulting in less frequent sexual activity; prostaglandin activity and perhaps hormonal factors. The more severe the endometriosis, the more likely there will be an infertility problem, although there are women with minimal disease and minimal symptoms who are infertile.

Because infertility often results as the disease progresses, and since endometriosis generally worsens over time, it may be important for those with the disease, especially those who want to conceive, to be treated as soon as the disease is diagnosed. However, because of the nature of current treatments, which are, for the most part, temporary (with the disease returning in time after treatment), and because the treatments themselves have risks, women without severe symptoms may choose to take a wait-and-see approach, deciding on no treatment or attempting a pregnancy before treatment.

It is generally recommended that pregnancy not be postponed if it is wanted, and the woman and her partner are ready to raise a child. Postponement could greatly reduce the chances of conception in the future.

However, we caution you not to forget that pregnancy is a *life* choice and not to rush into it simply because of fear of not being able to become pregnant later. Ways to "buy time" include treatments such as birth control pills or danazol to hold the disease in check as you make a decision about childbearing. Talking with women in your local Endometriosis Association chapter or support group or from the member contact list will also help greatly as many of them have faced similar situations. A counselor sensitive to women as whole persons, not just "baby-makers," can help you sort through the emotions and confusion that can arise when you learn you have a disease such as endometriosis.

When treatment is the choice, three types are available through traditional medical professionals—hormonal, surgical, or a combination of the two. (In addition, many women report to the Association that they are trying "alternative" treatments— nutrition, exercise, acupuncture for pain, chiropractic, homeopathy, and so on. The Association is compiling results on these and all treatments of endometriosis in its data registry.)

Hormone therapy for endometriosis usually attempts to simulate pregnancy (birth control pills) or menopause (danazol). Progesterone-based drugs are also sometimes used. All aim to stop the process of endometrial buildup and shedding, to bring about relief of endometriosis symptoms, and to dry up endometriosis colonies.

There are cautions in using hormonal treatments for women who want to conceive. If a woman becomes pregnant while on hormonal therapy, the chances for infant abnormalities now or many years from now, as with DES, are very real. Thus, danazol and the birth control pills are prescribed to be started at the time of your period to be sure you are you not pregnant. A nonhormonal method of birth control (such as diaphragm, or condoms and foam used together) is recommended while on danazol and progesterone. Reports to the Association indicate ovulation does continue for some women on hormonal treatments, particularly danazol. Because of the great emotional concern around pregnancy for many women with endometriosis, and the desire of many for pregnancy, no woman in this situation should take the chance of finding herself pregnant under conditions where termination of the pregnancy might have to be considered or continuation would occur under great emotional stress. Also, it is recommended that pregnancy not be attempted for a couple of months after hormonal therapy to give the body a chance to rid itself of the drug and to readjust hormonally in order to support development of a health fetus.

A final caution: progesterone-based drugs, according to *Womancare, A Gynecological Guide to Your Body* (see Recommended Readings), is probably an unwise choice for the woman planning a pregnancy soon after treatment. This is because progesterone-based drugs may suppress ovulation for long periods of time (ranging from months to years) after treatment and thus prevent conception.

Conservative surgery is another alternative open to women who want to bear children. Endometrial implants can be removed by cutting or cauterizing, adhesions removed, a severely damaged ovary and tube removed, and organs restored to their correct positions. Recently, laser surgery is also being used by a limited number of surgeons and is said to conserve fertility better than traditional surgery because less tissue is destroyed and scar tissue does not result. Also, danazol and surgery are being used together—with danazol used before surgery to dry up small growths, and after to dry up growths impossible to remove in the surgery.

Surgery may be the choice for a woman who wants to conceive who has large cysts, extensive adhesions, or pelvic anatomy distortions, which hormonal treatment would not be able to affect. Or, if a woman is older and feels she does not have the time to wait for months of hormonal treatment to continue attempting pregnancy, she may choose surgery.

A precaution with surgery is that, although a good surgeon will follow fertility surgery procedures to prevent adhesions, surgery itself can cause adhesions that could further contribute to infertility. Also, it is generally considered impossible to remove some endometrial growths with traditional surgery because of size (they can be microscopic) or location (if attached to the bowel or other vital organ or inaccessible). The latter can be removed with laser surgery or microsurgery in the hands of an expert surgeon, however.

Pregnancy rates following hormonal and surgical treatment of endometriosis are often debated and disputed and should be regarded skeptically until further data exist. Pregnancy rates following treatment with the birth control pill, for instance, range all the way from 5 percent to 73 percent; for surgery, from 38 percent to 87.7 percent; for danazol, from 15 percent to 75 percent.

Whatever the treatment, the extent of the disease and adhesions before the treatment are important factors in the pregnancy rate following treatment. Also, more pregnancies occur soon after treatments—the more time elapses from treatment, the less chance for pregnancy.

If a woman with endometriosis does conceive, will her pregnancy be normal? There is no easy answer to this question because very little research on the pregnancy experiences of women with endometriosis has been carried out. Generally, authorities say yes, with two exceptions: women with endometriosis have a higher rate of miscarriage and a higher rate of ectopic pregnancy (two problems that have been researched and documented), probably because of damage to the tube from the disease. (Ectopic pregnancy, you will recall, is a pregnancy in which the fertilized egg implants outside the uterus, usually in the fallopian tube.) This is a potentially life-threatening situation because, as the fertilized egg enlarges, it may rupture the tube and cause serious internal bleeding. Danger signs of a possible ectopic pregnancy would be a missed period in a month when conception was possible, with slight bleeding seven to fourteen days after the missed period, and mild soreness or pain at first with sharp pain later. Faintness, nausea, and vomiting might also occur, or shock. Help should be sought immediately.

Additional information on the pregnancy experiences of women with endometriosis became available through a study by Yale graduate nursing students Carolyn Ansell and Catherine Gorchoff. At the urging of the Association, they studied the complete pregnancy, labor, and postpartum experiences of women with endometriosis. A total of 187 members who had attained 334 pregnancies shared their experiences for the study. Ansell and Gorchoff found the women had multiple discomforts during their pregnancies, particularly nausea and vomiting; a high incidence of dysfunctional labor; high rates of postpartum depression; and a faster return of symptoms in those who did not breastfeed. (Write the Association to obtain more information on this study.)

If a woman with endometriosis conceives, what will happen to her endometriosis? In the past, pregnancy was often said to cure endometriosis, but now it is known that this stubborn disease returns far more often than not. Most reports to the Association indicate the symptoms (pain, etc.) disappear during the pregnancy, with recurrence after the pregnancy. The length of remission seems to be related to the severity of the disease, with a severe case recurring more quickly. A way to lengthen the time of remission is by breastfeeding—if ovulation is suppressed by the breastfeeding, the disease will usually stay in remission during that time. The most important factors are getting started right away after the birth, and breastfeeding the baby on demand without supplementary formula. Be sure to read materials on breastfeeding or check with the La Leche League or a similar group to learn how to breastfeed in the way most likely to stop ovulation. Two good books for breastfeeding and pregnancy in general are *Pregnancy and Childbirth: The Complete Guide for a New Life* by Tracy Hotchner (Avon, 1979) and *Nursing Your Baby* by Karen Pryor (Pocket Books, 1973).

There have been a few reports to the Association of the disease worsening during pregnancy, and medical authorities now believe the relationship between endometriosis and pregnancy is poorly understood. Early, repeated pregnancies were said, in the past, to protect against endometriosis, but that is also being questioned as women with such histories are found with endometriosis.

Becoming pregnant once does not assure further pregnancies. In a chapter summarizing medical thinking on endometriosis in the Obstetrics and Gynecology Annual 1981, it was noted that "only about 20 percent of patients who had coincidental pregnancy and endometriosis conceived again regardless of whether persistence of the disease was observed." Finally, good nutrition can play an important role in conceiving, with a high-protein diet and the B vitamins considered especially necessary.

By *Mary Lou Ballweg and The Endometriosis Association*

Sexually Transmitted Diseases

Over one million Americans each year fall victim to sexually transmitted diseases (STD). Defined as infections that pass from person to person usually through sexual contact, STDs can cause complications that lead to infertility in women.

Because STDs can range from mild to life-threatening, any woman who plans to become pregnant should first have a thorough physical examination. Not only will such an examination protect her from serious complications, if she does have an STD, but it will also protect her unborn/newborn child.

Be aware that many STDs are without symptoms; others are easily recognizable. Some STDs are peculiar to women; other affect both women and men. *All are contagious.*

STDs are unpredictable at best, and diagnosis can be uncertain. Some STDs — chlamydia, gonorrhea, and ureasplasma, for example, have similar symptoms but require different methods of treatment and different medicines. It is also common for one partner to exhibit symptoms while the other may not.

Sexually transmitted diseases, if undected or untreated, can cause infertility. Caution is essential. See your physician *before* attempting to become pregnant.

SECTION 3

Male Infertility

Introduction

For years, infertile women labored under the delusion that infertility was all their fault and suffered mental and physical anguish as a result. From biblical days, a woman who could not conceive was called barren, as if some part of her body was empty or missing. The Old Testament story of Sarah and Abraham is a case in point. Sarah, the reader will recall, was unable to conceive. Years of unsuccessful efforts to conceive passed; then when Sarah and Abraham reached a childless old age, Yahweh appeared to Sarah and told her that, indeed, she would conceive. Sarah thought the idea of conception at her age was so ridiculous that she laughed at Yahweh, but she did indeed conceive, and nine months later, Isaac was born.

At no time in this familiar story did anyone think that Abraham's sperm count might have been low.

There are a number of reasons for low sperm count including alcohol, marijuana, stress, and sexually transmitted diseases. Yet, men with a low sperm count *can* impregnate if the sperm are able to swim in a forward motion and at least 60 percent of the sperm are normal in size and shape. In this section, we will discuss male infertility, its causes, and how to cope with it.

Causes of Male Infertility

Fertility depends on several physiological events and their timing. The male partner must produce sperm of sufficient quality, quantity, and motility (swimming ability) to impregnate the woman. The woman must produce a healthy egg (ovum). Sperm is deposited in the vagina and then moves up through the cervical mucus to meet the ovum, which is still in the fallopian tube. Timing is important because the ovum lives for as little as twelve hours and no more than twenty-four hours; the sperm lives for one or two days.

There are a number of causes for male infertility:

1. Sperm production and maturation. Problems with sperm production and maturation may be caused by previous infections, particularly those that took place after puberty, such as mumps.
2. Undescended testicles.
3. Chemical and environmental factors and occupational hazards.
4. Sperm motility (movement). Sperm movement problems may be caused by chronic prostatitis (inflammation of the prostate) and low or very thick semen. Also, some drugs used to treat emotional disorders can affect the motility of sperm.
5. Conduction problems. These can be caused by scar tissue in the passageways through which the sperm travel or by infections or untreated sexually transmitted disease (STD).
6. Sexual dysfunction. Any of the following problems may be categorized as male sexual dysfunction: premature ejaculation— inability to control the ejaculatory reflex; impotence— inability to be aroused or to maintain an erection; dyspareunia—pain with intercourse; and sexual aversion—lack of interest in sex.

Impotence and premature ejaculation are causes of inability to deposit sperm into the cervix. Structural problems with the penis also account for this inability to deposit sperm in the cervix, i.e., when the penis opening is either on top or on the underside of the penis, rather than on the tip. Some neurological ailments and spinal cord injuries also prevent proper sperm deposit.

Sperm Ills Cause 40 Percent of Infertility

In at least 40 percent of the cases of infertility, the problem can be traced to the male partner.

During routine testing, urologists will evaluate sperm count, motility (spontaneous motion), and morphology (shape), all of which affect a man's fertility potential. We also check for any hormonal factors that may affect fertility and determine the temperature of the testes with a procedure called scrotal thermography.

Healthy sperm can be produced only when the testes are about two degrees cooler than core body temperature. In addition, we will routinely check the size of the testes, which reflects the ability of the individual to produce the sperm.

In 30 to 40 percent of the cases I've seen, the sperm count is low even though all other findings are normal. In these situations, referred to as idiopathic oligospermia, my colleagues and I treat patients with drugs to stimulate pituitary hormones on a three-to-four-month trial basis.

One common condition leading to male infertility is a varicocele, a collection of varicose veins that drain the testes, the glandular, sperm-providing bodies housed in the scrotum. In about a third of my male patients troubled by infertility, I find a varicocele to be the cause.

Normally, the veins are lined with one-way valves that carry blood in one direction. This mechanism prevents backflow. In a varicocele, the valves are missing, or the anatomy of the veins is such that a back pressure is created, causing a backup of blood. Most patients may be born without these valves within the veins.

While the physician can sometimes feel the bulging veins during a urologic examination, detection of varicocele may require the use of Doppler ultrasound, a machine that can pick up abnormalities in bloodflow through high-frequency sound waves.

Another diagnostic method that my colleagues and I use is called the isotope scan. With this sophisticated and painless procedure, radioactive isotopes are injected into an arm vein, and sensitive equipment registers the flow of isotopes through the scrotum.

In addition to directly observing the accumulation of isotopes, we are employing computer analysis to study the results of the scan. Once we determine the extent of varicocele and the degree of stasis, or stagnation, we decide whether or not to operate.

The correction is accomplished by simple out-patient surgery, and the procedure causes only minimal discomfort. The patients return to work within twenty-four to forty-eight hours.

With local anesthesia, we have utilized a "mini-incision" to perform the surgery with an operating microscope. With this technique we may effectively seal off varicose veins, and in my practice, the pregnancy rate following this simple procedure has been 35 percent.

Microsurgery is also used to reverse vasectomies for men who change their minds about wanting to be infertile. I have found this procedure to be successful 80 percent of the time, resulting in adequate numbers of sperm reappearing in the ejaculate. Other men with blockages, caused by infection and scar tissue, may be helped by microsurgery as well.

Finally, other new research is also playing a major role in the diagnosis and treatment of male infertility. In the laboratory, human sperm may be "washed" with nutrients and mixed with zona-free hamster eggs—eggs whose outer coats have been removed with an enzyme called tripsin.

These zona-free hamster eggs can accept sperm from any animal, including humans. Urologists can now actually witness the interactive process between sperm and egg and determine penetration scores. If the semen specimen can demonstrate penetration in at least 10 to 15 percent of the hamster eggs, it usually means that the patient has a pretty good fertility potential.

Probably the most useful spinoff of this research has been sperm washing in intra-uterine insemination. The washing technique replaces the semen with a nutrient solution.

The weak sperm and unwanted components, such as prostaglandins—chemicals that cause violent uterine contractions—are removed. The final washed preparation makes it possible to implant the sperm directly into the uterus.

With continued efforts in the areas of research, diagnosis, and treatment, our success rate with these patients can only go up. We try to coordinate our efforts with our gynecologic colleagues, and we try to tell these patients not to give up.

By *Dr. Joel Marmer*

The Case of the Reluctant Sperm

When a father-to-be appears to be in robust good health, it comes as a bitter surprise to discover that his sperm is not viable. Perhaps he needs to understand the factors that are preventing his sperm from making contact with his partner's ovum.

The testicles, placed safely in the scrotum, manufacture the sperm. The testicles are outside the body for a very specific reason: to keep the sperm cooler. Some men have, perhaps, noticed that the scrotal sac changes position as the weather changes, making it a natural thermostat to keep the temperature just right for sperm production. The last male bodily function to stop at death is sperm production.

Sperm maturation takes place in the epididymis, a tube that is almost twenty feet long. The epididymis connects with a larger duct, the vas deferens, familiar to most men as the duct where vasectomy takes place.

There are two semen sacs behind the bladder that emit a fluid that carries the sperm, and the vas deferens connects these vesicles in the prostate gland to form the ejaculatory ducts. The left and right ejaculatory ducts enter the urethra inside the prostate gland that surrounds the bottom of the urethra and adds an alkaline, milky fluid to the semen. The end product of this complex internal mechanism is ejaculated through the penis when it is stimulated.

Usually, a very small amount of fluid is expelled in a single seminal emission. In a fertile male, there are from 120 million to 350 million sperm per cubic centimeter in that emission. These athletic little swimmers can move very quickly up the uterus and fallopian tubes of the female partner and will usually stay alive for a few days.

The spermatozoa take a little over two months to form, and another two or more weeks of travel through the male reproductive system before they reach the ejaculate material.

What can make this intricate system fail? We know that 85 percent of normally fertile couples who attempt pregnancy succeed within a year's time, with 60 percent achieving pregnancy in the first three months of trying. In males, normal fertility means a sperm count of at least 20 million per cubic centimeter (the American Fertility Society disputes this and states 40 million per cubic centimeter is the minimum number of sperm), with 60 percent of the sperm structured normally, and with 60 percent also showing motility (movement) after ejaculation. Researchers believe that the normal form of the sperm and the vitality of the sperm are more important than the numbers.

The infertile male can have any one or more of the following sperm problems:

1. Less than 10 million sperm per cubic centimeter of fluid (*oligospermia*).
2. No sperm at all in the semen (*azoospermia*). When there is no sperm in the semen, it is not only important to check the testicles, but also the urine since, in some men, a problem in the nervous control of the bladder neck permits ejaculation into the bladder. It is also important to separate functional from pathological low sperm count.
3. Substandard semen (*dyspermia*).
4. No ejaculate at all (*aspermia*), which is usually found in nervous system disorders like syringomyelia (a disease of the spinal cord in which fluid accumulates in the cavities, replacing the nerve tissue and causing muscular atrophy and even spasticity), or paraplegia/quadriplegia.

The above problems usually result from other, deeper difficulties in the male physiology. It is easy to understand that spinal cord difficulties like those mentioned above are caused by accident or military action, but what about the other sperm difficulties? Why do they happen?

Varicocele

Varicocele is a varicose enlargement of the spermatic cord veins, and one of the most frequent causes of male infertility. It not only leads to reduced sperm but also to decreased sperm motility. Studies reveal that 80 percent of those with varicocele have abnormal sperm findings.

The varicocele can be removed through surgery with almost immediate improvement in the quality of the sperm. A study of patients who underwent surgery for varicocele revealed that, in 80 percent of the cases, the sperm quality improved,followed by a pregnancy rate of 50 percent.

Testicular Failure

The most common cause of testicular failure is aplasia (the defective development of the sperm-producing cells). This can be the result of a genetic defect, infantile or undescended testes, low gonadotropin (a gonad-stimulating hormone), inflammation of the testicles, tumor, injury, and radiation.

Treatment for testicular failure includes hormones such as clomiphene citrate, testosterone, and gonadotropin; however, these have had mixed results.

Duct Obstruction

Male infertility often results from obstruction of the ducts as a result of infection or surgery. The infection, usually caused by a sexually transmitted disease, commonly gonorrhea, but possibly tuberculosis, may be located in the epididymis (the small, oblong structure resting upon and beside the posterior section of the testes). The result of this infectious invasion is a blockage of the epididymis, and the resulting interference with sperm maturation. Other organisms responsible for infections that interfere with sperm are T-Mycoplasma and chlamydia Both are treated with antibiotics, including Dovacyclin and Vibramycin.

Autoimmune Conditions

When autoimmune conditions occur, the sperm becomes clumped (see Semen Analysis, this section). In some cases, this autoimmune response is because the male somehow produces an antibody to his own sperm. Corticosteroids have helped this condition, and the drug Dexamethasone helps in 40 percent of the cases. Dexamethasone, however, has many side effects.

Other Problems

Low sperm counts are caused by cytotoxic drugs (used to kill cancer cells). Cytotoxic drugs are most involved in causing azoospermia (absence of sperm in the semen).

When there is a congenital absence of the vas deferens, a low sperm count occurs. Vasectomy also involves this gland, but it is a deliberate surgical removal of all or part of the vas deferens. Since the inception of microsurgery, vasectomy reversals have improved. About 50 percent of males who have had vasectomies can, after reversal surgery, achieve pregnancy; however, it takes about six months before sperm production returns to normal. It is also important that reversal surgery be done within ten years after vasectomy. If more than a decade passes, the male often develops antibodies to his own sperm.

Caffeine and Sperm Count

Can caffeine make a man more fertile? Sounds ludicrous, but according to Dr. Joseph Barkay of Central Emek Hospital in Israel, the answer is yes. A decade ago, Dr. Barkay artificially inseminated fifty-eight women with five parts semen and one part caffeine. The result? Ten percent more of the women in the caffeine injected group became pregnant than in the control group, who were artificially inseminated with untreated sperm. Babies born to the women who received the boosted sperm were healthy and showed no chromosomal abnormalities.

Scientists, knowing that caffeine interferes with cell metabolism, began mixing caffeine with semen samples early in the 1970s.

New Yorker Dr. Cy Schoenfeld, the first to do test tube research on human sperm and caffeine, is reported in *Omni* magazine (May 1980) as saying, "Under the microscope, a perked specimen looks like the rush hour crowds in New York City subways. An unperked sample looks more like Sunday in the subways."

The possibility of pregnancy is higher when sperm is boosted with caffeine because it swims at double the ordinary speed; whereas, in infertile men, unfit sperm cannot make it to the ovarian tubes where fertilization takes place.

Semen Analysis

As part of any infertility workup, an analysis of the male partner's semen must be made. The man will ejaculate a sample of his semen into a clean container that must be kept at body temperature and examined quickly under a microscope to determine the number and movement (motility) of the sperm.

A normal sperm count is over twenty million sperm per cubic centimeter. Below ten million sperm per cubic centimeter is considered poor, although men with low sperm counts have been known to impregnate. At least 60 percent of the sperm should be normal in shape and size.

The sperm must be able to swim in a forward motion. Many men have difficulty begetting children because their sperm clump together rather than swim singly. When this social clumping occurs, the individual sperm cannot gather enough momentum to penetrate and fertilize the female's egg. Researchers believe that a vitamin C deficiency is a major cause of sperm clumping.

Because a man's sperm count can fluctuate, it is important that semen analysis be repeated at least once.

What to Do When Sperm Clump Together

Infertility researchers have discovered that men whose sperm clump together have a vitamin C deficiency. Taking this important vitamin in doses of one gram per day for a week is recommended. Vitamin C, also known as ascorbic acid, helps the body absorb important trace elements into the blood—zinc, copper, magnesium, potassium, and calcium. These trace minerals influence the independence and vigor of the sperm.

A 1983 study of 35 young men, in whose bodies clumped sperm measured much higher than the 25 percent figure researchers say marks the line between infertile and fertile men, all had low vitamin C levels in their blood. These potential fathers were given a daily supplement of one gram of vitamin C, and the problem dissolved quickly.

In one week, vitamin C levels in the blood and sperm of these young men were normal, and blood levels of the trace minerals increased. The sperm stopped clumping and also lived longer.

SECTION 4

The First Stairstep: The Low-Tech Approach to Fertility

Introduction

We've explored the major causes of infertility and, in some instances, reported the generally accepted treatment for the specific cause. Now, it is time to begin the Stairstep Approach toward solving the bigger problem of infertility that persists even when the cause has been eliminated.

A healthy body is, perhaps, the first step in the Stairstep Approach to healing infertility. To this end, "Healthy Pre-Conception and Achieving Pregnancy" is written by Barbara Feldman, director of the Fertility Awareness Center in New York City, who emphasizes a non-invasive approach to fertility that, in her own words, is "designed to give optimal health to both partners."

The emphasis on good health cannot be stressed too strongly, and Joy Gardner not only underlines the importance of optimum health but offers some natural remedies that can be of invaluable help to the non-fertile couple.

Working with Mother Nature is something that most people in our modern society have forgotten how to do. Dr. V. Virginia Vetrano offers the reader some important clues on how to become pregnant, with particular stress on fasting and what it can do to restore the body's health.

Suza Norton writes about the fasting process as a time of renewal and rest for body, mind, and spirit. She also offers pointers on how to begin to detoxify the body through fasting.

Herbs have helped many couples become fertile, and Susun Weed offers some fertility promoters that wise women over the centuries have found helpful.

Judé d'Amato presents an overview of non-traditional approaches to infertility. Her article not only discusses diet but also alternate treatments for infertility such as chiropractic, naturopathy, homeopathy, massage, and acupuncture.

Acupuncturist Ken Smith blends the "diagnostic and therapeutic benefits of traditional Chinese medicine with Western test results to design a course of treatment that can last anywhere from one to two cycles to a full year." His approach is different from what most Westerners have experienced; however, his high success rate with infertility (over 90 percent resulting in pregnancy) makes acupuncture a viable consideration.

Suzannah Cooper, a Fertility Awareness instructor, teacher, and author, gives readers a broad overview of infertility with all its pains and problems and explores a number of remedies that, in her experience, have proven effective.

Healthy Pre-Conception and Achieving Pregnancy

We live in an age and society where infertility has become a problem. Women in their thirties and forties are planning first babies when their chances of becoming pregnant are down, and birth defects are higher. New medical technologies are so complex that it's difficult for the average person to fully understand what is happening and to make informed choices about infertility treatments.

My work utilizes a non-invasive approach that's designed to give optimal health to both partners. With this foundation, conception, pregnancy, and birth become part of the life experience instead of a medical phenomenon. Having a child is a major responsibility. Having a child when you're older creates the additional responsibility of ensuring your own longevity and health in order to see that child through to adulthood.

My focus in pre-pregnancy counseling is on achieving pregnancy in the healthiest, most natural way possible. I meet with couples in a relaxed atmosphere for two hours or more in the first session. We focus on nutrition, their work environment, their relationship, and any emotional stressors. Together, we construct a health plan within the reality of their lives. I also teach them how to chart mucus and temperature fertility signs. One month later, we meet again to review this information and evaluate the next step.

Teaching the biology and nutrition of fertility is easy, but helping couples follow through to maintain motivation and willpower takes much more effort. I suggest that having a healthy pre-conception is as time-consuming—and certainly as important—as a full-time job. Some couples find the information overwhelming—at the very least, a threat to their life style. However, in time, many come to understand that a conscious conception begins with caring enough beforehand to create the healthiest conditions possible. In some cases, couples who require biological cleansing may have to delay pregnancy for six months to a year to better their health. In nature, a healthy seed in rich soil fed by a pure environment will produce a radiantly energized fruit. In human terms, the condition of sperm, egg, and mother all play a vital part in the potential pregnancy.

Instead of rushing into the high-tech medical route in fear and panic because you cannot conceive, consider a natural approach first. Depending upon the problem, there may be a self-help approach to reverse infertility in selected cases, even when you've been told that nothing can help but drugs and/or surgery. Recently, I worked with a woman who used alternatives (fasting, massage, and major dietary changes) while waiting to see the next specialist. During the six month waiting period, she became pregnant.

Natural methods can sometimes improve the quality of the sperm and semen, reverse the sperm/mucus allergic reaction, and reverse anovulatory conditions resulting from overweight and underweight. Because a man continuously produces sperm and semen, he can improve their quality in a relatively short time with better nutrition and the elimination of toxins like alcohol, nicotine, and other drugs. Sometimes, if he is continuously exposed to toxins he may have to change work environments. The woman with "hostile" mucus is more likely to provide the alkaline environment that sperm needs to survive by switching to an alkaline-based diet that consists of live fruits and vegetables. Most cooked foods, animal flesh, animal milk, and junk foods are acid producing.

Some natural methods to consider are fertility awareness, diet, fasting, and a happier and more relaxed life style. Specifically, fertility awareness is a means of appreciating the miracle of reproduction and predicting ovulation before it occurs. In medical settings, quick instruction on charting temperature is given without mentioning the more accurate sign of cervical mucus. Whereas temperature can signal ovulation once it has already occurred, the analysis of cervical mucus signals the ovulation event before it occurs.

The pre-conception diet should be as free from harmful substances as possible, ideally consisting of whole, live, organically-grown foods. Meat and milk should be eliminated because livestock, unfortunately, are given unhealthy feed with growth-stimulating hormones and antibiotics that can be detrimental to reproductive health. Often, the "calcium question" arises when a non-meat diet is suggested. With a reasonably low protein intake, high levels of calcium are not required, and vegetation is sufficient to supply human needs.

For most couples, these diet changes are quite difficult, so at the Fertility Awareness Center, we supply educational materials and contacts with others who've already made changes for the better. There are many creative ways to help people learn not to give in to food cravings or social pressures. My clients sometimes motivate themselves personally and politically by focusing on the larger issues that relate to vegan (no foods of animal origin) diets, for example, the need to preserve valuable rainforest land instead of turning it over to McDonald's for cattle grazing.

I also teach couples how to fast safely in order to reduce or eliminate toxins that have accumulated over the years. Change should be gradual, beginning with a vegan diet to minimize any problems associated with too rapid a detoxification process. The next step is a juicy fruit diet for several days, or, as some advocate, a raw fruit juice fast. Then, if one is psychologically and physically prepared, a pure water fast can follow, but only under supervision. You will need support and careful guidance for any type of fasting.

Light is also an important factor in reproductive health. Try to be exposed to at least fifteen minutes of sunlight a day without wearing sunglasses or contact lenses. Try to avoid artificial lighting as much as possible. Light exposure at night can interfere with the menstrual cycle.

Do find out if your tap water is safe to drink. If not, search for a source of pure water. Many potentially harmful chemicals are added to drinking water, and in some areas, pesticides pollute drinking water by seeping into the groundwater. Like the meat issue, water supply is related to environmental issues. In seeking fertility, you cannot help but become more conscious about the planet. Perhaps, in this process, you'll become active in supporting safe sources of energy and begin a recycling program in your home. Also be aware that many toxins can be found in deodorants, shampoos, cleansers, make-up, clothing, carpets, bedding, and building materials. Substitute natural products to reduce harm in your environment.

Other simple hints can make a difference: avoiding lubricants for lovemaking that can harm sperm, (for men) avoiding hot baths and saunas that can affect the quality of sperm, and experimenting with the frequency of intercourse to become pregnant (usually, couples are advised to limit intercourse to every two days or so, whereas some conceive only after making love twice in one evening).

Laughter and fun are healing for mind, body, and spirit. Even when you can't seem to conceive, you need to give yourself permission to laugh and be joyous and let go of so much seriousness. Many times, relaxation and fun require planning in busy life styles. Exercise also reduces stress and helps to eliminate toxins from the body. Stretching, aerobic, and weight-bearing exercises increase muscle tone, oxygen intake, blood circulation, and digestion. Exercise also calms emotions that can run high in couples who are frightened of infertility. The alternative healing practices—massage, meditation, relaxation exercises, and yoga—also have many health benefits.

In the wake of the fitness craze, you are flooded with advice to cut down on alcohol, red meat, and coffee. However, "The Moderation Myth" is misleading advice that says a little poison is O.K., which can jeopardize your pre-conception program. Since the egg and the sperm are minute individual cells, the belief (and teaching by health professionals) that undesirable elements, like coffee, alcoholic beverages, drugs, and toxic food, can be used safely in moderation, is, to say the least, misleading. A defect in DNA can be caused by very small amounts of toxic substances, and toxins accumulate in the body with constant, albeit moderate, abuse. The body's immune system, when so precariously imbalanced, can fall into toxic crisis with the added stress of a pregnancy which, in turn, can lead to miscarriage, stillbirth, or birth defects.

By *Barbara Feldman*

For further information contact her at the Fertility Awareness Center, P.O. Box 2606, New York, NY 10009.

The Effects of Lubricant on Sperm

In 1975, a research team investigated the effects on sperm motility of fifteen substances that could be used as vaginal lubricants. They found that the commercial vaginal lubricants were all spermicidal, and sperm motility decreased remarkably as early as fifteen minutes after incubation. Other substances, such as lotions, were also spermicidal. Although commercial vegetable oils (olive oil, safflower oil, peanut oil, petroleum jelly, and glycerin) decreased the sperm motility, none of them inhibited motility totally. Glycerin in as low as a 2 percent concentration immediately caused a slight decrease in sperm motility. It appears that all vaginal lubricants impair sperm motility and should not be used by infertile couples. Saliva has been recommended as a lubricant; however, it has been found that saliva impairs sperm motility and activity. Sperm motility and progression decreased significantly thirty minutes after incubation with as low as 2 percent of saliva. Higher concentrations of saliva significantly decreased sperm motility and progression as early as fifteen minutes after incubation. Furthermore, saliva induced a shaking movement (vibrational motion without forward movement) in 12 percent of the total sperm population incubated with high concentrations of saliva. These studies demonstrated the deleterious effect of all vaginal lubricants on sperm motility. Conversely, raw egg white has no effect on sperm motility and progression. Raw egg white might be considered as a vaginal lubricant for the small number of infertile couples who need it. Couples should be cautious, however, about the use of foreign protein substances in the vagina. Absorption of these materials, and the development of allergic reaction might occur. Additional studies in this area are needed.

From "Effects of Lubricant on Sperm" in *Medical Aspects*, February, 1986.

Being in Good Health at Conception

A major factor in the health of a child is the mother's health *at conception.* The father's health is also vitally important. As prospective parents, you would do well to exercise or do physical work outdoors each day; sleep enough so you don't feel tired when you wake up; don't overeat, and avoid refined foods (especially white sugar, white flour, and white rice); avoid junk foods and packaged foods made with chemicals, preservatives, and artificial flavorings, and eliminate coffee, cigarettes, and drugs.

Carrying a baby puts a strain on a woman's calcium supply, so have your teeth checked and try to get your dental work done before you conceive. If there are X-rays to be taken, make sure they put a protective apron over your abdomen. Don't have X-rays at all unless they're really necessary.

If you've been using birth control pills, wait at least three months before you try to conceive, because the changing hormone cycles can cause spontaneous abortions.

Maintaining Health and Fertility

There are things you can do to prolong your health and fertility.

Natural Birth Control

You should be aware of the possible long-term effects of contraceptives on your fertility. Birth control pills work by blocking the production of ovarian hormones, so that ovulation cannot take place. Some women who have taken the Pill for five to ten years have experienced reduced fertility, some have had no periods whatsoever, and some have been rendered sterile.

The IUD works by irritating the lining of the uterus so the fertilized egg won't implant. When the uterus has been irritated every month for a number of years, it can become difficult to conceive.

Condoms and diaphragms and the Ovulation Method are non-invasive methods of birth control which will not affect your future fertility.

If you are healthy and don't smoke, drink, or use drugs, and you observe the following regimen, beginning in your thirties, you can hope to maintain the optimum health of your reproductive organs and hence your fertility for far longer than the average woman.

Dong Quai and Fasting

Dong quai (also spelled dom kwai or tang kuei; the Latin is *Angelica sinensis* or *Angelica polymorpha*) is primarily a Chinese herb, the female counterpart of ginseng. It contains plant substances that are similar to female hormones, and it is used to strengthen and restore the female organs. Dong quai is not generally recommended for use during pregnancy or for women with excessive menstrual flow. It is popular in China for restoring the female organs after childbirth and for easing the changes of menopause. This is an excellent herb for regulating the periods. It is used for purifying the blood and strengthening the circulation. You can buy the whole dried root at herb stores, including Chinese herb stores.

One of the best ways to take dong quai is in combination with fasting. Ideally, set aside one to two weeks (or at least two or three days), preferably in the spring or autumn, and try to fast or eat a simple diet (just fruits and vegetables, for example). During this time, drink plenty of teas and/or juices, including two or three cups of dong quai tea per day.

Dong Quai Tea. *Boil 6 cups of water in a pot. Then, add 1 medium or large root. If you like, add about 1 tablespoon of licorice root, about 1/2 inch of cinnamon stick, and 1 tablespoon of fresh grated ginger root. These other herbs are health-giving, and they add flavor to the tea. Simmer for at least 20 minutes, replacing the water as it evaporates.*

You can begin such a program of fasting and drinking dong quai tea at the age of thirty, once a year, and after thirty-five, twice a year—unless you are in poor health or have smoked more than ten cigarettes a day for over a year, or otherwise abused your body, in which case you might do it as frequently as four times a year, until your health is restored.

If you cannot fast, take dong quai occasionally, especially when your periods are irregular or more uncomfortable than usual. Nibble off a pea-size piece of the root once or twice a day (if you prefer, you can prepare tea and drink one or two cups per day). Do this for three to ten days before your period is due. Depending on your health, you may want to do this every month, or just a few months per year. Another way to maintain your fertility is by strengthening your endocrine glands.

Difficulty Conceiving

According to Dr. Robert Kolodny, coordinator of the Masters Johnson Reproductive Biology Research Foundation, one out of every eight couples in the U.S. has difficulty conceiving. In at least 40 percent of these cases, the situation is caused either wholly or partly by low sperm production.

If you are having trouble conceiving, consider your health, your habits, and your environment. You and your partner should both see a doctor to determine if you are in good health. The man should have a sperm count taken. When you're quite certain that you want a child, and if you're in good health, you will probably get pregnant soon with the following methods. If you try these methods conscientiously for three months without results, consult a doctor who is a specialist in fertility.

Regulate Your Periods and Determine Your Fertile Days

If your periods aren't regular, it's difficult to anticipate your fertile days. So the first step is to try to regulate your periods.

Dong Quai

This Chinese herb is the female equivalent of ginseng, which is well known as the longevity and virility herb for men. Dong quai contains plant substances that are similar to female hormones. It's good for the female organs, though it should not be taken during pregnancy. Dong quai can be purchased at most herb stores, including Chinese herb stores. Usually, it is sold as a dried root. Nibble off a pea-sized piece of the root twice a day. Your period will probably become regular within a month or two. Then, you will probably need to continue taking the herb for three to ten days before each period is due. After you stop using birth control, discontinue using this herb.

Lunaception

This is a method of regulating your menstrual cycle. It is based on the observation that the light-sensitive pineal gland, which is located in the central part of the brain behind the "third eye," plays a role in regulating ovulation. Many years ago, Louise Lacey did some research which suggested that before the advent of electricity, women had "moon cycles"; that is, they ovulated and menstruated in relation to the full and the new moon. Ms. Lacey speculated that electricity has thrown off women's menstrual cycles.

I was interested in her theory, because I noticed that women who live in rural areas (away from city lights) often menstruate at the same time, usually at the new or full moon.

Perhaps it is the stimulation of this gland by light which explains why farmers can induce chickens to lay more eggs by putting a light on in the chicken coop at night.

Louise Lacey found a study conducted at the John Rock Reproductive Clinic for infertile women in which women slept with a one-hundred-watt light on the floor at the foot of their beds for the fourteenth, fifteenth, and sixteenth nights of their menstrual cycles, counting the first day of their period as day one. They found that previously irregular, infertile women were able to regulate their ovulation cycles into a regular twenty-nine-day rhythm, ovulating predictably on the fourteenth or fifteenth day. They experimented with using the light on various other nights, but found that only this formula worked effectively. Ms. Lacey noticed that this rhythm followed the same pattern as the moon cycles, with the light bulb mimicking the nights that the moon was full or nearly full.

Experimenting with herself and eighteen friends, Louise Lacey found that they could regulate their monthly menstrual periods. They also found that by using this method, their periods kept perfect rhythm with the new and full moons—except when they were under severe stress. She found that this method could be used effectively both for getting pregnant and for birth control. (She cautioned that Masters and Johnson found that there were some highly fertile women who sometimes ovulated when they had an orgasm. She said that these women would notice irregularities in their charting, and that this method of birth control would not work for them.)

Here is the method.

1. Prepare your bedroom. Ordinarily, it is essential to sleep in complete darkness, so you may need to buy heavy drapes or a shade, or put a cloth along the crack at the bottom of your bedroom door. Then you will need a low power light source, such as a fifteen-watt night-light, plugged into a socket near your bed, or a forty-watt bulb in the closet, or a dim hall light to use three nights a month. It should not be bright, but it should be perceptible through closed eyelids.

2. Make a chart. Buy quarter-inch-ruled graph paper. Position it so that the long side runs from left to right. On the far left column, leave two blank lines at the bottom and then, moving upward, write a list of temperatures, by tenths, going from 97.5 degrees Fahrenheit, and then on the next line up, 97.6 degrees, and then 97.7 degrees, and up to 100.0 degrees at the top.

Along the top, one to a square, list the dates, starting with the date you began using the chart. You may want to wait until the end of your current menstrual cycle.

3. Take your temperature daily. Buy a good-quality oral thermometer. Don't buy the cheapest, regardless of guarantees, because the temperature needs to be exact, and the cheap thermometers are not reliable. Decide on a time of day when you will take your temperature. The important thing is to do it the same time every day, within about fifteen minutes. If you get up early during the week and sleep in on the weekends, it might be more reliable to do it around dinner time. Do not smoke, eat, drink, or brush your teeth for ten minutes beforehand. Leave the thermometer in your mouth, under your tongue, for at least four minutes (this may not be relevant with a digital thermometer). If you have a cold or other infection, or are under severe stress, your temperature may not be normal. So you need to chart your temperature for at least three months before you can be sure of a pattern. Make a dot on the graph in the column below the date, exactly opposite the temperature the thermometer shows. Draw a line from

one dot to the next.

4. Use the light. You will need to know what day the moon is full. Many calendars indicate the time of the full moon, or you can get an astrological calendar. Count the day of the full moon as day fifteen, and then on the nights of days fourteen, fifteen, and sixteen, sleep with your light on (if you live in the country where there are no artificial lights, just leave your curtains open). On all other nights, sleep in a darkened room. (If you live in the country, you can still leave your curtains open.) Within a few months, you should be ovulating with the full moon (however, some women menstruate with the full moon and ovulate two weeks later with the new moon).

5. Read the chart. When ovulation occurs, there is a change in your hormones which will be reflected in your daily temperature. There will be a slight fall, followed the next day by a steep rise of as much as a whole degree or more. This is called a phase shift. The temperature will then stay high, varying as much as a full degree up or down, until the next period, when it will fall back to the original temperature. When your period becomes regulated with the light, the phase shift will occur predictably the night before you sleep with the light on.

While a phase shift covers a period of forty-eight hours, ovulation takes only a few seconds, and the fertility of the egg lasts for about eight hours. Since you cannot know which eight of the forty-eight are fertile, you should take advantage of the whole period. Also, sperm can live for forty-eight hours inside a woman's body, so if you are using this as birth control, you should abstain from sexual relations or use some other form of contraception for at least a full five days—two days before you use the light (before the anticipated phase shift) and the three days you use it. Do not rely on this as a form of contraception until your cycles are reliably regular. The only really safe way to use this method is to wait until you have definitely ovulated, and then wait another three days after that. Before ovulation you can use another form of birth control.

The Ovulation Method

This is another method for determining your fertile days. It can be used in conjunction with Lunaception, or it can be used separately. It is also used for birth control. The Ovulation Method is based on the knowledge that estrogen increases in a woman's body until it reaches its peak, at which time another hormone, luteinizing hormone, is released, causing an ovum to erupt from the ovary and to begin its journey down the fallopian tube, where it can be fertilized. At this time, the rise in estrogen level causes the os (the mouth of the uterus through which the sperm must travel to reach the ovum) to open up. During this time the ovulation mucus stretches itself into a corridor pattern that leads the sperm directly up to the uterus. These corridors vibrate within the same frequency range as the tails of the sperm! The ovulation mucus is richly supplied with glucose to nourish the welcomed sperm, so that they may live and fertilize for as long as five-and-a-half days.

Ovulation mucus not only enhances the possibility of conception, it is a prerequisite for it. After ovulation, the tacky, sticky cervical mucus sets in and the os closes up. Then, the cervical mucus blocks the cervix and the closed os with a cobweb pattern of mucus which helps prevent the sperm from getting through. This kind of mucus is high is leukocytes (white blood cells) which surround the sperm and ingest them. It also contains anti-trypsin. Trypsin is an enzyme in the head of the sperm which enables the sperm to break down the outer shell of the egg and enter it. Finally, this mucus also contains factors which tend to clump the sperm and stop the movement of their tails. Most sperm cannot survive more than a few hours in such an unfriendly medium.

The challenge, then, is to learn to identify the ovulation mucus. There are two kind of secretions in a healthy woman's vagina: the secretion produced in response to sexual stimulation, and the cervical mucus which comes down from the cervix (the neck of the uterus). Just before ovulation, this cervical mucus resembles egg white; it feels slippery and it can be "stretched" without breaking. To test this, insert your index or third finger slightly into your vagina and get some mucus on your finger, then touch your thumb to the mucus and slowly move your thumb away from your finger. The mucus should stretch out in long strands between the two fingers. You may notice this slippery mucus when you wipe yourself after urinating.

After observing your mucus for a full cycle between periods, you'll become aware of the changes it undergoes. You can learn to identify the ovulation mucus and then, if your observation is correct, the menstrual period will begin eleven to sixteen days after the ovulation mucus becomes most stretchy. Since semen closely resembles the consistency of ovulation mucus, instructors ask women to abstain for one month before using the ovulation method in order to observe their mucus without confusion.

This method works even if your periods are irregular, or if you are coming off the Pill, or if you have just had a baby. By observing the mucus each day, you can tell when you are ovulating. This method should be used in conjunction with the charting described under Lunaception. Each day you can mark on the chart whether your mucus is tacky or slippery.

If you want to use the Ovulation Method for birth control, it is strongly recommended that you find an instructor. Classes usually involve a two-hour presentation with follow-up about a month later. To obtain the names of teachers in your area, send a self-addressed, stamped envelope to The Ovulation Method Teacher's Association, P.O. Box 14511, Portland, Oregon 97214.

Strengthen Your Endocrine Glands

Vitamins A and E. These vitamins are necessary for the optimum health of your endocrine glands, which regulate ovulation and influence sexual energy. Both the man and woman should take 10,000 I.U. of vitamin A and 800 units of alpha tocopherols each day. Fish liver oil, which is one of the richest sources of vitamin A, is a time-honored remedy among native people for women who are having difficulty conceiving.

Licorice and Sarsaparilla. A tea made of these herbs will strengthen the woman's endocrine glands. Drink one or two cups per day. Store in the refrigerator. You can drink it cold. It is a pleasantly sweet drink.

> ***Licorice and Sarsaparilla Tea.*** *Boil 6 cups of water and add 2 tablespoons of each herb. Simmer for 20 minutes and then strain.*

Acupressure

In Chinese medicine, the kidney meridian governs the sexual energy. The end of a meridian is a powerful point. The kidney meridian ends at the center of the ball of the foot; it will be tender at that spot. With your thumb, press firmly at this spot while making a clockwise movement. This (or almost any other form of pressure) can be repeated on each foot for up to three minutes every day. Several women who had trouble getting pregnant conceived within a month after using this pressure point. Don't hesitate to try it; there's no harm done if you get the wrong spot.

Effective Positioning

This method usually works for women who know when they ovulate. The idea is to place your uterus in the optimum position to receive the sperm and then give the sperm ample time and the assistance of gravity to reach their destination. This is especially effective when the man has low sperm production or low sperm motility.

For one week before you expect to ovulate, don't have sex, but do flirt. This makes the sperm strong and concentrated and makes the woman more receptive.

On the day of ovulation, do not drink any liquids because you will not be able to urinate for a long time after intercourse. You should be sure to urinate before having intercourse.

Lie on your back with your knees up toward your chest. This facilitates deep penetration and helps to create a pool of sperm around the cervix. After the man ejaculates, he should gently withdraw his penis.

Then try to maintain the same position for as long as possible—more than four hours is best. You can put your feet up against the wall and have your partner pile cushions under your legs and all around you. Arrange to have a good book, television, and music nearby. It's O.K. to eat, but avoid salty foods because you don't want to drink. Avoid liquids because you don't want to urinate. If this method sounds quite impossible because you tend to urinate frequently, consider placing an incontinent pad or diaper under you.

Try to repeat this procedure again after twenty-four to thirty hours (but not sooner), and again after forty-eight to sixty hours. It usually works the first month, but don't give up until you've tried for two or three months.

By *Joy Gardner*

Want a Baby? Let Nature Help

Life just doesn't seem fair. Some people who don't want them have babies while others yearn for them and can't have them. In the past, adoption was the only alternative. Fortunately, there are other alternatives today, but none are comparable to having your own baby. How would you like to be able to have your own baby? How would you like to be so fertile that you had to be very careful or you *would* get pregnant? Such cases happen very frequently when you resort to living according to the laws of Nature.

Fasting (water only), followed by correct eating and living practices, often increases fertility to such an extent that pregnancy frequently occurs when it seemed impossible before.

After coming back to my health school for a second supervised fast for asthma, my patient told me how she immediately became pregnant when she got home after her first fast. Laughingly, she said she and her husband call it their "hygienic baby." They already had raised one family, now here's a new one! They weren't unhappy but, on the other hand, they had not expected or planned for any more children. Pregnancy, after fasting on water only, happens so frequently that those who don't wish to become pregnant must be extra cautious after a cleansing fast. So you see, conception is within your reach simply by understanding and heeding the laws of physiology.

Many women (men also) who are not fertile become so after detoxifying the "fast" way. If a woman is unable to conceive, the fast is often the very thing that will enable her to do so. If she desires to bear children, there is every reason for the human female to trust in Nature and, by fasting, to put her tissues in the most healthful state possible. It is the most natural way to cleanse the system. Furthermore, fasting not only is harmless but also extremely beneficial in all ways. Both domesticated and wild animals use fasting instinctively when injured or feeling out of sorts. It is part of the total way of life for all living beings on this planet.

The reason why fasting enables the female to conceive is because enervation (chronic fatigue) and toxicosis impair the function of every organ and tissue in the body. Hormones in the healthy individual are maintained in a very precise balance. They must be secreted in exact quantities and in proportion to the demand made by another hormone or the target organ. Too much or too little of any of the female hormones can mean the difference between ovulating or not ovulating. This is the reason why the Pill can prevent ovulation. Likewise, toxicosis interferes with the precise regulation of the female hormones. In addition, when toxicosis prevails, the female secretions become lethal to the sperm, and the sperm cells succumb before reaching the ovum. In these cases, fasting is a sane and harmless means for achieving pregnancy. Medicating or drugging the vaginal tissues, while occasionally enabling a woman to conceive, does not remove the cause of the abnormal secretions, and frequently harms the baby. Only a truly natural way of life and fasting can be of lasting benefit in these conditions. When the baby finally comes, it has a greater chance of being normal and exceedingly healthy if no drugs were used before or during pregnancy.

Some conditions that decrease fertility, but are often remedied by fasting and right living, are female eunuchism, tumors of the uterus or ovaries, abnormal function of the genital system (birth defects, etc.), hypogonadism causing a failure to ovulate, salpingitis (inflammation of the fallopian tubes), endometritis (inflammation of the lining of the uterus), low grade inflammation or infection of the cervix, and abnormal hormonal stimulation of the cervix. Infection or inflammation of the cervix and an abnormal hormonal stimulation of the cervix can lead to a viscous mucus plug that will prevent fertilization. Many of the foregoing problems are effects of endocrine imbalance, and most of them are completely remediable by hygienic means.

The uterus and its inner lining, the endometrium, are frequently the site of new growths of various types. Tumorous masses in and around the uterus may affect fertility in some way. If one has a tumor of the uterus and conceives, the tumor is likely to grow, especially leiomyomas (fibroids). Besides, it interferes with the normal function of the uterus and could be a detriment to normal delivery and to the nourishment of the growing fetus.

Consequently, it is best to fast away tumors of all kinds as soon as one is discovered. If you wait too long, the tumor may become so large that surgery is necessary; whereas, if you fast as soon as possible, you prevent its becoming larger, and you won't have to fast so long to absorb it. At the same time, you will be achieving another end—that of detoxification. Your endocrine system, indeed your whole body, will function better, and you will have gotten rid of the cause of your tumors. Thus, the re-growth of tumors is less likely. If they are cut out, your uterus becomes scarred and less able to withstand pregnancy and parturition. Additionally, *surgery does not detoxify the body.* On the contrary, surgery fills you with many unneeded medications and wastes nerve energy, leaving you more prone to the development of tumors in the future and less able to bear healthy children. Fasting permits your body to absorb the tumor, cleanse itself, and ready itself for normal reproduction.

While fasting, the body breaks down nutrient matter previously stored for future use at times of accident or scarcity. It takes from less-needed organs and tissues in order to supply the more vital organs with nourishment. Consequently, you do not starve while fasting because your body is living off its stored reserves. Tumors are absorbed because the body considers them more expendable than heart, lung, or muscle tissue. The size of the tumor, its blood supply, and the type of tissue of which it is composed, determine how rapidly it will be absorbed. If the tumor is very large, you may require more than one fast.

Most inflammations, including salpingitis, endometritis, cervicitis, vaginitis, etc., cause abnormal secretions. Depending upon the severity of the condition, they don't always cause infertility, but they do predispose to it, especially when it is of long standing and severe. Wherever there is inflammation of the genital organs, the secretions of that area become more or less abnormal and can destroy the sperm. Long standing salpingitis causes fibrosis and blockage of the fallopian tubes. Then, the ovum cannot make its way through the tube and dies before becoming fertilized. Once toxicosis is eliminated by fasting and correct living habits, fertility improves. Fasting of sufficient length causes the various inflammations and abnormal secretions to subside. While fasting, the body casts out mucus plugs as well as some fibrous tissue. Extraordinary results are observed by fasting under the supervision of someone who is knowledgeable in natural hygiene.

It is best to have lived according to the laws of life for at least a year before becoming pregnant. If this seems too long for you, then take a good cleansing fast first, get plenty of rest, and wait a month or two, then conceive. By fasting and living properly before conceiving, you will be in a better condition for pregnancy. If you have properly prepared your body, you won't develop morning sickness, toxemia of pregnancy, varicose veins, hemorrhoids, or lose your teeth, or any other problem supposedly associated with pregnancy. In fact, you will hardly know you are pregnant, except when your baby undulates in your uterus. If you are infertile and the problem is serious, you may need two or three fasts before you can conceive. Getting rid of the serious conditions permits the body to detoxify. You will, therefore, automatically achieve the health necessary for an easy pregnancy and parturition.

To show you the extraordinary remedial effects that accrue from fasting, I'll tell you about a young actress who was infertile because of hypogonadism. Actually, she was a female eunuch. This twenty-six-year-old's breasts were undeveloped, and her uterus was still infantile. She was extremely tall, a characteristic of female eunuchism. This pathological condition causes the long bones to continue growing for a longer time than normal; consequently, affected females are very tall. Besides being infertile, she was anorexic. She seemed to fear eating, so she would eat nothing all day long and end up glutting at night. Being extremely thin and tall, she looked like a walking skeleton. When she became uncomfortable from overeating, she frequently caused herself to vomit.

In spite of all the emotional problems, she was a wonderful, fun-loving young woman who desperately wanted to have children and get over her anorexia. She was already underweight when she consulted me, and fasting necessitated losing more weight. This made it difficult to give her only one fast of sufficient length for her complete recovery. Rather than one fast, she had a series of fasts on water only.

It may sound strange that a person who is too thin to start with should be fasted. However, when conditions are desperate, sometimes it is necessary; nevertheless, it is safe. As astounding as it may seem, thin people fast very well. They handle the fast with greater ease than some heavier people, and they often lose weight much more slowly, so their reserves last longer than you would think by looking at them.

Her first fast was for twenty-six days. This was followed by a completely uncooked diet composed of fresh vegetables, fruits, nuts, and seeds. She was still anorexic, but at least when we fed her, she began eating in the daytime. She spent several months at the institution, eating and living in accordance with physiological laws. She went to bed early, exercised regularly, rested in the afternoon, enjoyed sunbathing, and relaxed in the fresh country air. In other words, she wanted to get well so much that she was willing to do everything possible to recover. After regaining some weight, she took her second fast, which was two weeks. Again, she went on the uncooked diet, not taking any medicinal herbs or spices. This was the ultimate in permitting the body to heal itself.

She was given instructions to follow when she returned to her home in New York. She meticulously followed instructions at home, securing her sunshine, rest, sleep, maintaining emotional poise, and eating correctly while, at the same time, pursuing her goals. She found a man she loved and married, not even thinking that she could have children, because her physician told her she was undeveloped and had hypogonadism. Although motherhood was desirable, she fasted and began living correctly, more for her emotional problems than for her fertility. Nature is generous; give her what she needs, and she will reward you in multitudinous ways. This young woman did not realize what her body could do when freed of its toxic load and given its needs. Toxicosis inhibited the function of all the cells and organs in her body. Like her, very few people realize the powers of the living organism until they are proven.

These organic capabilities were proven to my patient when she conceived. She began to develop normally, even after an age when development should have ceased. Her uterus became normal in size. Her breasts and other secondary sexual characteristics developed, and she became a whole, normal human female capable of all the functions Nature intended for her. It was a wonderful and enlightening day when she gave birth to a beautiful baby girl and, later, to a sturdy, healthy boy.

If fasting can heal such deep-seated endocrine problems as hypogonadism, I am certain that you can have faith that correct living and fasting will help others who have less serious conditions.

Fasting is of benefit in cases of internal and external endometriosis. This is a very serious fertility disorder which may be helped only if the problem is caught before too many abnormal tissue changes have taken place. Endometriosis is one of the most common causes of female sterility.

If not remedied at its inception, so much fibrous tissue is built up in the abdomen that it causes great pain as well as irreversible sterility. The scar tissue often grows and covers the ovaries, encapsulating them. Thereafter, the ovum is prevented from reaching the fallopian tubes, where it normally would meet with its mate to form a new, wonderful creature. If fasting is instituted in the early stages of endometriosis, all the fibrous tissue that might build up over the years can be avoided, and the woman will be able to conceive. If just a small amount of fibrous tissue has been deposited, and the individual fasts to eliminate toxins, the secretions and excretions of the vagina and endometrium become normal, and the woman may become pregnant. Endometriosis (internal and external) must be prevented rather than treated. After the condition has been allowed to last so long that the ovaries are surrounded and enshrouded with masses of scar tissue, it may be too late.

The ideal way to avoid all female problems is to be reared hygienically, or at least to put hygenic principles into practice at an early age. Endometriosis develops most often in women in their third and fourth decades. Since there is a higher incidence of this condition in women who marry late and who tend to have fewer children, it, like breast tumors, seems to develop not only because of living habits, but also because of failure to utilize all our natural physiological abilities—namely, having babies.

To safeguard yourself from all female problems, it is necessary to secure all of the requisites of physiology, such as pure water, fresh air, natural foods to which we are biologically adapted, equanimity (poise of the mind), sunshine, and congenial friends. Additionally, it is necessary to avoid all enervating, poisonous, and toxic substances, such as coffee, teas of all sorts, chocolate, processed foods, condiments, alcoholic beverages, soft drinks, smoking, etc. In other words, provide the conditions of health and avoid the causes of disease, and you can't help yourself—you will be healthy in all ways.

Getting back to my opening statement, "Life just doesn't seem fair," let me assure you that it is much fairer than you may realize. You simply have to know the rules. From infancy on, we are educated to mistrust our instincts. Over the centuries, science led us to believe that we can, without penalty, tamper with natural bodily processes. We were led to believe that it is actually beneficial to "regulate" and "influence" physiological processes. Regardless of whether or not we are hungry, we are urged to eat. When we are sick, we are told we must eat to keep up our strength. When we are well, we force feed ourselves for fear we won't be securing all the vitamins and minerals we've been taught we *must* have every day. When we are sleepy, we are made to believe we need a "pick-me-up" in the form of some cola drink or herb tea, coffee, tea, etc., instead of sleep. When we are frustrated, instead of thinking the matter through to find its cause and eliminating it, we get drunk, resort to some sort of drugs, or gorge ourselves on tempting morsels.

Perhaps it is time to renew our faith in Nature's wisdom. We must realize that there is much more to understand than the tip of the iceberg we already know. Nature is as fair as she can be, but when we constantly violate all the laws of life, we must accept the consequences of those violations. Law and order exists in the physiological realm just as it does in the physical, chemical, or any genuine science. If we trust our instincts more, and our medical or health education less, we will soon learn the laws which govern us. We can live in such a fashion that we will not become sick. We must learn to obey the laws of life.

The primal law for health, longevity, and fertility is to supply the body with the needs of life. By supplying these requisites of life, we avoid the development of those severe pathological conditions that prevent fertility, such as scar tissue from endometriosis or salpingitis. An additional benefit of right living is that your health extends to your progeny. Your children will be born with fewer tendencies to endocrine disorders. They will have fewer inheritable fertility problems.

In short, by living healthfully in the first place, one avoids the pathological consequences of disobedience. If one has not known what it is to live in accordance with natural laws and is faced with infertility but desires motherhood, then Nature and natural laws are still the best way back to health. They are still the shortest road to superior health and fertility, but remember that where natural law prevails, ignorance of these laws does not abrogate the consequences. If you are now faced with pathological developments that prevent fertility, complete reliance upon Nature and natural law should be your first resort. If you are confronted with infertility because of endometriosis or some other pathological development which may or may not be considered remediable according to the medical mind, it is still worth giving hygiene a first try. Hygienic care is not harmful. It is beneficial for complete well-being and superior health, not just for fertility. It produces no untoward side effects. The effects of right living are not ephemeral, but lasting, and go deep into your underlying tissues. Lastly, Nature surprises you. You may not think that you are becoming whole again by right living because it is not like medication; you don't see the effects immediately. But lo and behold! If you persist in living in accord with natural laws, one of these days you may suddenly find yourself healthy and happily pregnant.

By *Virginia Vetrano, D.C.*
For further information, contact her at Rio Frio, Texas 78879.

The Fasting Process

"Most of what we eat is superfluous. Hence, we live off only a quarter of all we swallow. Doctors live off the other three-quarters."

from an Egyptian papyrus

With some basic prior knowledge, you can make a fast or cleansing diet a time of rest and renewal for the mind, body, and spirit. An uninformed endeavor can easily turn into a depressing time of just dreaming about food, worrying that you're starving, not knowing why you waver between nausea and elation, and ending with gorging yourself all at once on the food you passed up. Volumes have been written on the body's need for a time of cleansing, and there are dozens of schools of thought about the best way to proceed. I won't try to give you the last word on the subject, but I will offer what I have found most useful and practical after looking in many directions.

Perhaps the most important prerequisite for a successful fast is moment-to-moment awareness. Many a hopeful cleansing attempt has been broken in a moment of distraction and/or weakness. (Believe me, I speak from experience!) How many times while absentmindedly eating too much rice pudding have our minds pretended that this will be the last bite—tomorrow for sure we'll live on salads and juices. Such a simple discipline as putting aside past memories and expectations of taste and satisfaction, letting go of future ideals, and bringing our senses into the present while munching Tamari Chips, is good mental preparation for a successful fast. The eternal conflict between what actually is (reality) and what should be (future ideal) is certainly exemplified in our eating patterns.

How Fasting Heals the Body

The secret of the curative effects of fasting and cleansing practices lies in the fact that the body, in its wisdom, will begin to decompose and eliminate those cells and tissues which are damaged and diseased. During a prolonged cleansing regime, you literally place your body on nature's operating table, as the body begins releasing toxic materials, tumors, abscesses, fat deposits, etc.

While you are on a cleansing program, the capacity of the eliminative organs—lungs, liver, kidneys, and skin—is greatly increased, and masses of accumulated wastes and toxins are expelled. The rate at which these toxins are expelled depends, I believe, on a person's health and body chemistry, and on the type of program followed (that is, just plain water, raw juices, all raw fruits and vegetables, cooked nonstarchy green vegetable soups, or a monodiet, such as brown rice). Many types of fasts and diets initiate a cleansing process, but some work more efficiently than others, and some apparently work better than others for certain people.

This eliminative process is evidenced by the following typical symptoms (intensity of the symptoms depends on the type of fast or diet used and on one's current state of health): bad breath, dark urine (the concentration of toxins in the urine can be ten times higher than normal), generous elimination from the colon (with the help of laxative herbs, cleansing juices, and/or the use of the controversial enema), skin eruptions, smellier than usual perspiration, and mucus discharge.

I found the chapters on fasting in Paavo Airola's *Are You Confused?* fairly sensible. Airola says he has supervised both water fasts and a combination fast of juices, herb teas, and vegetable broths, and considers the latter far superior. He reports the work of Dr. Otto H. F. Buchiner, who supervised over 80,000 fasts, and found this fasting method resulted in a much faster recovery from disease and was more effective in every way than a water fast. Airola gives the following justification for juice fasting:

1. Raw juices and freshly-made vegetable broths are rich in vitamins, minerals, trace elements, and enzymes. These vital elements are very easily assimilated directly into the bloodstream, without putting a strain on the digestive system. They do *not* disrupt the healing and rejuvenating process of autolysis (self-digestion of diseased, damaged cells and tissues), as has been suggested by some water-fast proponents.

2. The nutritive elements from the juices are extremely beneficial in normalizing all body processes, supplying needed elements for the body's

own healing activity and cell regeneration, and thus speeding recovery.

3. Raw juices and vegetable broths provide an alkaline surplus, which is extremely important for the proper acid-alkaline balance in the blood and tissues, since blood and tissues contain large amounts of acid during fasting.

4. The generous amounts of minerals in the juices and broth help to restore the biochemical and mineral balance in the tissues and cells.

5. Accumulative poisons such as DDT are released into the bloodstream during a fast. Fasting on juices and broths release DDT and other toxins more slowly into the bloodstream than a plain water fast, and these poisons are both better neutralized and more efficiently eliminated because of the high mineral and vitamin content of juices. Airola also recommends enemas, exercises, deep breathing, and other practices as needed to ensure a safe, health-giving fast.

(Many nutrition writers speak of the dangers of too many toxins being released too quickly into the bloodstream, especially when a person is already weak and in ill health.)

People who favor juice fasting over water fasting believe the main difference between the two is that, during the juice fast, the body's eliminative and detoxifying capacity is increased, and the healing processes are speeded up, causing you to feel far less debilitated.

Basics on Beginning a Fast

Basic, general advice is to prepare yourself for fasting by a short, cleansing diet. For two or three days, eat meals of the best-quality fresh fruits and vegetables available in your area. (In general, keep these meals simple, not mixing the fruits and vegetables.) People living in cities should find a source for unsprayed sun- or tree-ripened fruit. Many nutritionists warn that fruit which has been picked too early may contain undesirable acid. If good fruit is not available, use vegetables; learn to grow all kinds of sprouts on your kitchen counter. Ann Wigmore's books show how even city dwellers can have an abundance of organic, living, fresh greens readily available.

Use the best-quality water available for making herb teas and vegetable broths, and for diluting fruit juices. If possible, find a source for fresh vegetable juices; if you do not have a juicer, look into borrowing or renting one from a friend. There are many books that give specific programs, but use your intuition. Generally, it's best to use your own home-grown sprouts, celery, parsley, etc., rather than the gassed and wax-coated fruits and vegetables in the supermarket.

The ideal would be to fast in a situation where you are not tempted by food, with people who have fasted before and who can give you confidence. I have fasted under many different circumstances, and for me it works best if I can arrange my life so that I can be doing the things I enjoy most and can be quiet and rest when I like. If you have not successfully fasted under your normal living circumstances, it would be well worth it to put yourself in a situation more conducive to fasting.

By *Suza Norton*

Food intake has long been associated with reproductive health. Indeed, to menstruate, an adolescent girl must reach a critical weight of at least eighty-five pounds because fat tissue helps store estrogen, an ovarian hormone involved in the menstrual cycle. Also, cholesterol is a precursor to estrogen formation, so lowering cholesterol intake, as recommended to reduce the risk of heart disease may, in time, affect a woman's fertility. In Miracle Babies *(see Recommended Readings), Dr. Mark Perloe and Linda Gail Christie say that rigorous dieting can threaten fertility because it leads to nutritional imbalance, lowers the proportion of body fat, and causes stress. Perloe also cautions against a strict vegetarian diet, having observed cases where fertility returns once fish and eggs are added (provided there is no other problem). Yet, there are also intelligent arguments for using fasting as the means of eliminating accumulated toxins that contribute to infertility, and vegetarianism—when foods are combined to yield complete proteins—is now accepted as a healthy way of life. It's wise, in any case, to be guided by experts before attempting a fast.*

Fertility Promoters

The reasons for infertility are complex and differ greatly from woman to woman and couple to couple. Despite these complexities, I have found that it is often amazingly easy and straightforward to establish a pregnancy with the help of herbs.

Herbs used to encourage a pregnancy are characterized by their ability to: 1) nourish and tone the uterus; 2) nourish the entire body; 3) relax the nervous system; 4) establish and balance normal functioning of the hormonal system; and 5) balance sexual desire.

Red Clover Flowers

The single most useful herb for establishing fertility is *Trifolium pratense*. Its high vitamin content is especially useful for the uterus; its high protein content aids the entire body; its profuse and exceedingly absorbable calcium and magnesium relax the nervous system and promote fertility; its high mineral content, including virtually every trace mineral needed by the glands, helps restore and balance hormonal functions. In addition, red clover alkalinizes the body and may balance the acid/alkaline level of the vagina and uterus in favor of conception.

Red clover is in the pea/bean family. Add fresh flowers to salad. Cook a handful of dried flowers in with your rice. Red clover is often combined with peppermint in fertility brews, since mints are safe and pleasant-tasting sexual stimulants. Infuse one ounce of red clover blossoms and a teaspoon of peppermint (or any other mint) in a quart of water for four hours. This infusion may be taken freely throughout the day and for several months continuously. Alfalfa is regarded as a substitute for red clover, but I do not find it as effective.

Nettle Leaves

The common stinging nettle, *Urtica dioica*, is a uterine tonic and general nourisher with a special ability to strengthen the kidneys and adrenals. Its high mineral and chlorophyll content makes it an excellent food and tonic for the hormonal system. These characteristics make nettle infusion my second favorite brew for increasing fertility. As with red clover, drink one or more cups of the infusion daily for several months.

Red Raspberry Leaves

All *Rubus* species, but most especially the wild ones, provide leaves which contain an effective uterine tonic and a large amount of calcium. Raspberry leaf is my third choice as an herbal fertility promoter. It is most effective when combined with red clover. One or more cups of the infusion (prepared by steeping one-half ounce red clover blossoms and one-half ounce raspberry leaves in a quart of water for four hours) can be taken daily and continued for months. Another way to increase the fertility-promoting ability of raspberry is to add five to fifteen drops of either dong quai root tincture or false unicorn root tincture to each cup of raspberry leaf infusion.

Dong Quai Root

I have found *Angelica sinensis* invaluable in normalizing menstrual periods. It is widely and highly regarded as a fertility promoter. The form I favor is a water-based combination extract sold in Chinatown stores under the name "Tang Kwei Gin." Best results are obtained when dong quai preparations are taken during the days between ovulation and menstruation and discontinued from the beginning of the menstrual flow to ovulation. If the "Gin" is unavailable, substitute a homemade dong quai/comfrey root tincture. *Caution*: Use dong quai only in combination with other herbs.

False Unicorn Root

Chamaelirium luteum is regarded as a powerful and positive uterine tonic. It is also believed to have a strong beneficial and alkalinizing influence on the ovaries, kidneys, and bladder. Always noted as "the" herb for infertility, false unicorn root is difficult to obtain except in commercial combination tinctures and capsules. Dosage of the tincture is five to fifteen drops per day. The infusion is taken in sips, up to half a cup daily.

Lunaception

Ovulation is controlled by light. Leave a light on in your bedroom for three nights midway through your menstrual cycle; all other nights, keep the room in total darkness. You will ovulate when the light is on. Have intercourse during the three "light" nights if you want to conceive. This method, called *lunaception,* combines well with herbs which promote fertility.

PABA

Carlton Fredricks reports low levels of para-aminobenzoic acid (PABA) in women who have difficulty in conceiving, and increased success in conception with supplements of PABA, but does not give dosage information.

Calcium and Magnesium

Calcium and Magnesium are the two minerals thought to be the most important in affecting a woman's ability to conceive and maintain a pregnancy.

Vitamin E

There is a well-established link between vitamin E and fertility. Vitamin E is said to have a "dramatic" effect on the reproductive systems of both men and women. Five hundred to 1500 I.U. taken daily by the male partner for several months prior to conception has been shown to prevent birth defects in children of couples who had defective children. Wheat germ oil is my favorite natural source of vitamin E.

By *Susun Weed*

Egg Whites and Infertility

Odd as it may seem, several babies have been born to so-called infertile couples who substitute egg whites for their regular vaginal lubricant. Petroleum jelly and commercial gels destroy or inhibit sperm, but egg whites do not. Egg whites are made up of pure protein and actually facilitate the sperms' swimming action. There are no negative side effects from the egg whites. They are natural, inexpensive, and may be applied with any vaginal applicator.

Eating the Vegetarian Way

In the previous pages, infertile couples have been told how important it is to maintain optimum physical health if they want to have children. In recent years, eating a vegetarian diet has become popular in the United States, but can a vegetarian diet provide optimum health?

Vegetarians come in several mind-sets. There's the vegetarian who opts for a diet that eliminates red meat and poultry but includes fish, eggs, and dairy products, along with vegetables and fruits. Such a person is following a meatless diet.

The ovo-lacto vegetarian eliminates not only meats and poultry from the diet, but also fish; however, dairy products are included in the diet, along with fruits and vegetables. The vegan, by far the strictest vegetarian, will not eat any food from animal sources but eats an assortment of grains, fruits, seeds, and vegetables.

A carefully prepared vegetarian diet can be nutritious, perhaps even more so than a "regular" diet. The only nutrient that might be in short supply is vitamin B12, which has its source in animal products. A supplement may be needed.

Other nutrients are abundant in vegetarian foods. Protein is found in peas, beans, soy milk, grains, nuts, and seeds. Giving up cow's milk does not mean shorting the body of calcium because dark green vegetables, tofu (soybean curd), and fortified soy milk provide ample calcium. Vitamin D, given to us so generously in sunshine, is also added to most cow's milk. It is found in fortified soy milk as well.

Iron-rich foods are abundant in vegetarian diets and include whole grains, legumes, molasses (particularly blackstrap), and dark green vegetables.

Weight watchers may find a vegetarian diet to their liking because getting enough calories is a concern, not cutting back on calories. Of course, if one chooses ovo-lacto vegetarianism, then the problem of too many calories may remain because dairy products are high in fat—and calories. Plant foods, however, are much lower in fat than animal products.

Many people worry about getting enough protein in a vegetarian diet. Researchers insist that Americans usually ingest too much protein rather than too little; however, it is important that the essential amino acids are present in the diet. Most vegetable foods lack some of these essential amino acids, and so the vegetarian needs to learn how to combine vegetable foods so that one food provides what the other lacks.

This is not as difficult as it may sound. One combines, for example, a grain (rice, wheat, oats, corn, etc.) with a legume (lentils, dried peas, beans, peanuts) and gets not only a delicious food combination, but all of the essential amino acids. Is there anyone in the world who doesn't like a peanut butter sandwich? If the peanut butter is spread on whole wheat bread, all of the essential amino acids are present. Snackers can munch on roasted peanuts and sunflower seeds, or they can sprinkle some delicious sesame seeds over pea or lentil soup and, in both instances, they will provide their bodies with all of the essential amino acids.

Eating a vegetarian diet may not, of itself, assure fertility, but it can help to bring the body to optimum health and sustain it in top condition.

Non-Traditional Approaches to Infertility

Once the cause of a fertility difficulty has been established, there are various modes of treatment available. Some of the more traditional methods of treatment for males include administering steroids to treat low motility of sperm, male hormones for low sperm count, artificial insemination for low sperm counts which are motile, surgery for a blocked passageway or varicocele. Interestingly, statistics indicate that for the most part, males do not seem to respond very favorably to treatment.

Some of the more traditional methods of treatment for females include injections or oral administration of female hormones when there is a failure to ovulate or implant; antibiotic and/or steroid irrigation for tubal adhesions or blockages or for PID (pelvic inflammatory disease); and surgery (most often recommended) for uterine adhesions, polycystic ovaries, cervical problems tubal adhesions, and PID.

If a couple chooses not to follow a conventional mode of treatment, they may seek a more natural course. If this is the case, a naturopath, chiropractor, herbologist, homeopathist, physiotherapist, massage therapist, or acupuncturist may guide them to the proper therapy.

A general detoxification may be the first step, since accumulated toxins can interfere with any of the body's functions. This may include cleansing the colon with herbs, colon irrigations, or foods that will act as "brooms" for the intestines. Flushing the liver (the body's largest detoxifying organ) with a combination of lemon juice, olive oil, and garlic may be a tremendous detoxifying aid. Once the body has eliminated a lot of built-up toxins, better nutrition is provided to the cells. In many cases, this alone will allow the body to reproduce because it is being furnished with nutrients previously bypassing vital cells. Two of the nutrients essential to supply an environment for fetal growth are calcium and magnesium; some of the nutrients for proper liver function (since the liver is quite important for appropriate endocrine functioning) are riboflavin, thiamine, amino acids, and vitamin C. Often nourishment in the form of fresh vegetable and fruit juices is the most assimilable approach; and combinations of carrot, celery, spinach, beet, mung bean sprout, cucumber, apple, and citrus fruits are recommended. Sometimes vitamins and minerals are recommended in the form of food supplements. Recently, the availability of Spirulina, a microalgae plankton, has been found very useful because of its complete amino acid content, high vitamin A (carotene), B12, chlorophyll, and trace minerals.

To ensure that the body is fully utilizing the vital elements it is getting, it is necessary to investigate other areas of the body's functioning. For instance, if the spine and pelvis are not in alignment, nerves may be impinged, inhibiting organs and gland function. Therapeutic manipulation is frequently needed to correct this, and may take the form of spinal adjustments, massage, deep connective tissue therapy, polarity, or invasion therapy. In addition, there are many other signs that a qualified therapist can identify and evaluate when doing body work: tender flex areas can often indicate where the imbalances and weaknesses are, so that stimulating these areas with reflexology (pressure-pointing on the feet) and polarity can produce a favorable effect, to the point of correcting the condition. Specific attention should be given to the hormonal glands, particularly the pituitary—the "executive" of the endocrine system. Some of the herbs that act as special food for a woman's endocrine glands include licorice root, red raspberry leaves, squawvine, false unicorn root, and dong quai. Particular combinations of these herbs, either powdered and capped or made into an extract (for convenience and concentration), have proven especially effective. Ginseng seems to be the most effective herb for the male hormonal system.

If the problem is a tubal or uterine blockage or adhesion, an effective treatment appears to be castor oil packs applied to the lower abdomino-pelvic area. In some cases, alternating with packs over the lower back accelerates the process of breaking down the deposits to clear an open channel. A general routine can be worked out on an individual basis as to frequency and length of time for each pack, depending on the degree of the blockage or adhesion. This, combined with pressure-pointing reflexes (especially in the feet and buttocks) has cleared many blockages.

The length of time for response differs with the individual; it can be as short as two months or as long as nine. When working with some of the natural therapies, it is necessary to bear in mind that nature keeps her own pace and the human body's condition is rarely spontaneous. Thus, it takes some working with it to improve it. Nevertheless, in the midst of all the frustration, despair, isolation, helplessness, guilt, anger, and resentment that can emerge from infertility trauma, it's important to remember that there are many alternatives and solutions available. All it takes is a commitment to seek them out and patience while working at ameliorating the situation.

If you and your spouse are seeking these alternatives, begin by checking with doctors who are nutrition-minded. Many chiropractors will fall into this category or will be able to direct you to a qualified therapist.

By *Judé d'Amato*

Combining Eastern and Western Medicine in the Treatment of Infertility

Under his treatment philosophy, Ken Smith blends the diagnostic and therapeutic benefits of traditional Chinese medicine with Western test results to design a course of treatment that can last anywhere from one or two cycles to a full year. This depends on the severity of the infertility problem. To diagnose and treat Western as well as Eastern infertility syndromes, Smith does an initial workup that relies upon semen analysis, BBT charting, post-coital test, and hysterosalpingogram. "Many clients," explains Smith, "have already been tested extensively and come with records in hand."

Smith's interest in specializing in infertility came about somewhat by chance. While maintaining a general practice and treating a wide range of illnesses, he found many of his patients becoming spontaneously pregnant during treatment with acupuncture and herbs. This occurred even though he was not treating them specifically for infertility. They may have had a fertility problem in the past and, in assuming that they were infertile, failed to even mention this during the initial workup. Smith reasoned that, if pregnancy could happen spontaneously, how much better his results would be if he went to China to study with the top experts in the field.

"In the treatment of infertility with traditional Chinese herbal medicine," says Smith, "we have a complete system of medicine with a recorded history of infertility texts dating back over two thousand years to the Han Dynasty. Even at this early date, ancient Chinese physicians observed that infertility could be a male problem as well as a female one. Treating infertility is never easy by any method, and the Chinese approach is quite complicated and involved."

Smith quickly points out that he treats unique individuals and not necessarily syndromes. Although he may see ten different women who wish to become pregnant and who have a long miscarriage history, he may give each one a slightly different prescription that more suitably addresses her unique mental and physical state at that moment. (He has some patients who have had successful pregnancies after more than ten miscarriages. These patients required a course of treatment for six months to a year, making sure pregnancy did not occur during this time, as the herbs work to strengthen and restore the body's natural reproductive function.)

The Chinese believe that many cases of miscarriage are due to the couple having intercourse while pregnant. Sex during this time exhausts the energy of the kidneys, which are responsible for retaining the fetus. (Intercourse can exhaust a woman's essence as well as a man's.) Chinese doctors always advise couples to abstain for the first three months of pregnancy. If there are no complications, the couple may have intercourse, only very occasionally, for the remainder of the term.

Smith may continue to adjust a prescription to reflect the changing state of the patient as treatment continues. This is determined by feeling the pulse, which is the main method of diagnosis in traditional Chinese medicine. Felt on the radial artery, it comprises a minimum of twelve distinct positions with as many as twenty-eight different qualities, each of which has a particular clinical significance to the practitioner, who then composes a prescription for the patient, much like a composer writing a symphony. A highly experienced practitioner can actually write a precise, accurate prescription based solely on pulse diagnosis, without ever asking the patient a single question.

Smith has high success rates (over 90 percent resulting in pregnancy) in the areas of ovulatory failure. Other syndromes that respond especially well with Chinese medicine (80 to 90 percent) include hostile cervical mucus, luteal phase defects, frequency of miscarriage, low sperm count, poor motility, poor morphology, agglutinization of sperm, and excess or deficient volume of semen (either extreme can be a cause for infertility). Men with low sperm counts have traditionally had very poor results with Western drug therapy, with little hope in sight. Chinese herbal medicine is especially effective in this area. Treatment in this regard is also unique; not only are there herbal prescriptions to drink as a tea, but some special herbs are given to be eaten before bed. Smith comments that the taste of these herbs is actually sweet. He is currently developing an herbal "candy" bar for more convenience.

Immunological factors are another area with extensive research being done in China with the development of a formula called "Protect Antibody Soup." This prescription is unique, as both partners drink the same herbs while continuing to enjoy sex. It has a success rate of 65 percent. Sexual dysfunction can also be treated quite effectively with traditional Chinese medicine. Impotence, frigidity, and "sexual incompatibility," with one partner having excess sexual drive while her/his mate manifests a lack of desire, are commonly seen at the clinic. Smith urges great compassion and understanding here, as most cases are energetic in nature due to a hyperactivity or hypoactivity of kidney function and not due primarily to psychological factors.

Some of the more difficult cases to treat with a poor prognosis are those requiring surgical intervention such as poly-cystic ovarian disease, varicocele, blocked fallopian tubes, and endometriosis. In observing over six thousand clinical cases in China, Smith has never seen a case of endometriosis, "the career woman's disease," in a Chinese resident. All cases were from overseas Chinese, or those who traveled from Hong Kong or Macau, where a western-oriented, stressful way of life was evident.

One of Smith's greatest areas of success lies, ironically enough, in that of "unexplained infertility," where there is no known cause and all Western test results are normal. Here, the traditional Chinese medicine theory falls into the realm of two distinct syndromes: 1) "Liver Chi Congestion," and 2) "Tian Qui Deficiency" (Tian Qui" is similar to FSH or Follicle-Stimulating Hormone in Western medicine). The liver, in Chinese medicine, controls the emotions and nervous system. When congestion arises, energetic blockages develop in the reproductive process, thus causing infertility. This congestion is often due to a stressful life style.

Liver Chi Congestion often presents many symptoms like P.M.S. (Pre-Menstrual Syndrome). One symptom is irregular menstruation which varies, sometimes occurring early, and sometimes occurring late. Other symptoms can include the following: menstrual flow which is not smooth, sometimes starting and then sometimes stopping; dark colored blood with small clots; breast pain with distension (sometimes the distension can actually be observed); fullness of the chest; emotional swings, ranging from a melancholy depression to irritable fits of rage; nervousness; worry, and frequent sighing. Pulse diagnosis reveals a wiry and small pulse, sometimes accompanied by a slight irregularity in the pulse rate often likened to a "light knife scraping bamboo." Smith reports that results here are often dramatic. He has had some patients conceive within a single month of treatment.

In Tian Qui Deficiency, a minimum time of six months of treatment is needed before conception is attempted. One symptom here is irregular menstruation but, unlike Liver Chi Congestion, which can vary from being early to late, this is usually fixed, being one or the other. Other symptoms include: scanty or excessive bloodflow with a light, pale color and a thin blood consistency, and pain in the lower abdomen after menstruation is finished. The patient may also complain of tiredness, dizziness, palpitation, and weakness of the extremities. The facial complexion is yellow or pale. Chinese pulse diagnosis reveals a small, soft, sunken, and forceless pulse. This category often applies to women over the age of forty who are attempting pregnancy. Smith reports pregnancies in women up to the age of forty-seven. He will not, however, attempt to treat post-forty women unless he feels that they are strong enough energetically, and that there is a good chance of success for a full term pregnancy. He can determine this through pulse diagnosis on the initial visit.

"Patient compliance," explains Smith, "is very important for the efficacy of treatment." Some patients may not like the taste of the usually bitter herbs, or perhaps a busy life style makes preparation difficult. (Smith has easy-to-take pills available as well as freeze-dried herbal prescriptions but warns that, in severe cases, the boiling and drinking of the herbs may be the only effective treatment.) Time is also a factor, as treatment can take several months, during which time the couple may be asked to deliberately avoid attempting pregnancy (and, in some cases, also limiting the frequency of intercourse) in order to allow the reproductive system to regulate and strengthen itself.

Upon acceptance into Smith's program, a patient will be advised regarding possible life style changes, along with special diets and exercise recommendations. For patients who must travel great distances, he has a program requiring only one visit a month for acupuncture treatment and herb prescription evaluation. Smith predicts that Chinese herbal medicine will be offered in many of the infertility clinics located across the country.

This will help augment and support those programs, especially in the areas of unexplained infertility, low sperm count, and poor motility.

For further information contact Ken Smith, C.A., 3335 Mission Drive, Santa Cruz, CA 95065 or 279 South Beverly Drive, Suite 728, Beverly Hills, CA 90212.

Before Going to the Doctor

Infertility is on the rise, affecting as many as one in five couples. With fertility clinics springing up across the country, couples are undergoing a barrage of infertility tests and procedures, ranging from post-coital sperm tests to having radioactive dye injections, all in the hope of bringing forth a new life. Yet statistics indicate that much of this intervention may be unnecessary.

A recent review of studies on infertility shows that the majority of infertile couples eventually achieve pregnancy without medical help. Dr. Polly Marchbanks of the Center for Disease Control in Atlanta, Georgia reports that, in one study of 1,200 couples who were considered infertile because they could not conceive in two years of unprotected intercourse, 73 percent of them eventually became pregnant without medical help.

In another study, 84 percent of couples who had been unable to conceive after one year of trying were able to achieve pregnancy without help. Of 250 couples for whom biochemical causes of infertility were found, 72 percent were eventually able to conceive, taking up to ten years in some instances.

These data suggest that many of the interventive—and expensive—infertility tests and procedures can be avoided by couples willing to give themselves time to conceive. As a Fertility Awareness instructor, I have known numerous couples who, after years of unsuccessfully trying to conceive (often with the aid of extensive infertility procedures), finally become pregnant—after taking a few common sense steps toward understanding the factors that may have contributed to their infertility problem.

As with any health concern, no single remedy will work for everyone. Some may conceive only after undergoing extensive medical procedures. However, it seems prudent to consider simple, self-help measures before resorting to more interventive ones.

Taking Responsibility

The first step toward solving an infertility problem is to learn about your own natural reproductive processes. Rather than focusing on textbook theories and diagrams, you can learn how to check and chart your choice of three simple fertility signs: cervical mucus, basal body temperature (BBT), and cervix changes. These simple signs change cyclically in response to hormonal changes and offer a concrete way of documenting highest times of fertility and possible causes of infertility.

The majority of infertility clinics recommend BBT charting as the primary means of determining the time of ovulation. The woman takes her temperature daily, upon waking, and charts it on a graph. Temperatures are low before ovulation and higher afterward. A sustained BBT rise of three or more days usually confirms that ovulation has occurred.

However, once an egg is released from the ovary, it has only a twelve- to twenty-four-hour lifespan during which to become fertilized. This twenty-four hours is usually over by the time the third sustained BBT temperature occurs. In other words, *a woman charting BBT alone is informed of ovulation only after it occurs.*

Cervical mucus offers a great deal more information. The woman checks her mucus daily by wiping the labia with her fingers and records the kind of discharge that is present. When fertile, a woman has wet mucus. When infertile, she experiences dryness or an infertile-type mucus. Wet mucus helps sperm survive in a woman's body for three to five days and also signals impending ovulation. A woman becomes fertile as soon as mucus secretions appear following (or during) her period; ovulation then occurs at the end of this fertile buildup, anywhere from two days before to two days after the last day of fertile mucus (also known as "peak day"). Charting mucus changes in conjunction with BBT can increase the chances of conceiving by documenting times of highest fertility each cycle and indicating when ovulation is likely to occur before it happens. Changes in cervix position and quality confirm the information provided by mucus and BBT changes. When fertile, the cervix feels soft and high up in the vagina, and the os (opening) feels dilated. When the fertile mucus patch is over, the cervix feels firm, lower in the vagina, and the os is more closed and filled with a thick, infertile mucus plug. Ovulation marks the point of highest fertility in each cycle. It is easier to become pregnant if ovulation occurs before the fertile mucus ends, since sperm survival is increased by the mucus. If ovulation occurs after this, the timing of intercourse becomes crucial. With no fertile mucus present to help the sperm survive until ovulation, a couple interested in conceiving must have intercourse on the day of ovulation. (Sperm survive only a few hours when no fertile mucus is present.)

A Chart Example

In the chart example on the following page, the woman had her period, followed by several dry days. Her fertile mucus buildup then began with sticky mucus, becoming more creamy, slippery, and wet toward the end of the patch. She then experienced dryness (no mucus) for two weeks, until her next period arrived. (This two-week "luteal phase" is constant in all women.)

For the optimum chance of achieving pregnancy, a woman and her partner should have intercourse every other day or so when fertile mucus is present, and on at least two of the "post-peak" days (the first three days after peak day, during which ovulation might occur.) In this example, the temperature peak occurs on day fifteen, followed by three days of sustained readings over four-tenths of a degree. This indicates that ovulation most likely occurred before the fertile mucus patch ended. This couple would have a good chance of becoming pregnant, since fertile mucus would help the sperm from intercourse on days fourteen and sixteen survive in the woman's body until ovulation.

In this example, the temperature peak occurred on day fifteen, *after* the fertile mucus stopped. This is when timing becomes crucial. If ovulation occurred on day fifteen or sixteen in this chart (as the BBT indicates is likely), the egg could be fertilized only within its twelve- to twenty-four-hour lifespan. No fertile mucus is present to help the sperm survive in these post-peak days, so the woman literally has only one day this entire cycle during which she can become pregnant.

To achieve pregnancy when ovulating on day fifteen or sixteen in this cycle, then, the couple needs to have intercourse on the *exact* day of ovulation, since the sperm will die hours after lovemaking (with no fertile mucus present to extend their life). Therefore, having intercourse on days

KEY: ☐ = fertile ■ = infertile ▨ = bleeding

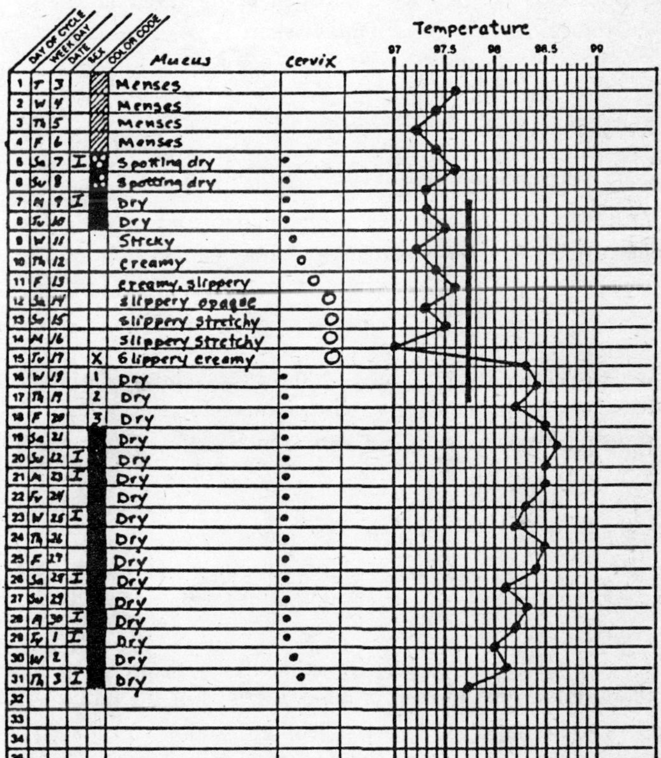

one and two post-peak ensures the couple the highest chance of achieving pregnancy when ovulation occurs after the fertile mucus ends.

Many couples who have been trying for years to conceive discover that their problem is simple one of timing. After charting mucus and BBT together, they learn that ovulation has been occurring *after* the fertile mucus stops, and that they have not been having intercourse during these first few transitional dry days. Timing intercourse to coincide with ovulation greatly increases the chances of conceiving.

Other Fertility Impediments

Many self-help techniques are available to couples willing to explore and alter some life style patterns which may be contributing to the difficulty in conceiving. The following factors can all affect fertility.

Diet

The consumption of refined foods, excess sugar, caffeine, or food additives can impede the liver's ability to metabolize hormones. If the liver is processing a great amount of these dietary substances, in addition to breaking down pesticides and other toxins, it will not break down estrogen and progesterone as efficiently. This can cause an extended fertile mucus patch, an insufficient luteinizing hormone surge (the hormone which triggers ovulation in response to a drop in estrogen at the end of the fertile mucus patch), and delayed ovulation. Eating a well-balanced diet of whole foods can resolve this problem.

Because infertility has been linked with a suppressed immune system, it is also a good idea to test for food allergies or intolerances that may weaken the immune system. Applied kinesiology is a reliable, noninterventive way to test for allergies; other approaches include a microwave radiometer, a RAST test, or a food rotation/elimination diet.

Vitamins

An imbalance of vitamins and minerals can cause a hormonal imbalance and interfere with fertility. Nutrients in sperm include calcium, magnesium, zinc, sulphur, and vitamins B12, C, and inositol (part of the B vitamin complex). Lack of these substances can lead to low sperm counts, lack of semen, and lowered sex drive.

Vitamins B, C, and E, as well as magnesium, manganese, zinc, and lecithin, help the woman's body properly metabolize cholesterol, which is needed for the production of estrogen and progesterone. Excessive or insufficient amounts of these nutrients can interfere with mucus production and delay ovulation. A zinc deficiency, in particular, is said to be responsible for many infertility problems in both men and women. The safest option is to avoid extended use of vitamin megadoses (more than 400 to 500 percent of the US-RDA recommended levels) and to nutritionally correct any extreme vitamin or mineral deficiency.

Amount of Body Fat

A 17 to 21 percent amount of total body fat is necessary for good health and proper hormonal functioning. Ovulation can occur only when estrogen rises and drops, triggering a surge in LH (luteinizing hormone), which then causes the release of the egg. Too little or too much body fat can interfere with ovulation by causing estrogen levels to be either too high or low to trigger a sufficient LH surge.

Estrogen (which causes fertile mucus) is formed from cholesterol in the body. Progesterone (which causes infertile mucus) is produced from estrogen. A woman with too little body fat (such as a long distance runner or anorexic) is unable to produce sufficient estrogen to trigger ovulation. Her mucus chart would reflect this condition by showing only a few days of scant, sticky mucus in lieu of a normal fertile buildup, with a light breakthrough bleeding instead of a period. Increasing dietary intake of some unsaturated fats can remedy this.

Obesity, or too much body fat, produces excessively high levels of estrogen, which the liver must then break down. This can prevent a sufficient LH surge and thus inhibit ovulation. Excessive estrogen causes longer fertile buildups, delayed ovulation, and irregular cycles.

Contraceptive pills utilize this principal by creating a synthetic hormonal imbalance: The high-estrogen contraceptive pill prevents ovulation by producing an estrogen level too high to trigger the LH surge, the progesterone "mini-Pill" allows ovulation to occur but creates a hostile uterine lining, which prevents the fertilized egg from implanting. In a similar way, obesity may lead to miscarriage—by producing too much progesterone and thus interfering with implantation.

Mucus charts accurately reflect hormone levels. An extremely long fertile buildup with a great amount of slippery, egg white type of mucus indicates high estrogen levels; infertile mucus that is creamy, rather than sticky or dry, also indicates high estrogen levels. To reduce estrogen levels for proper hormonal functioning, determine your optimal body weight and strive to achieve this by balancing a whole-foods diet with daily exercise.

Light Pollution

The pituitary gland, in conjunction with the hypothalamus and pineal glands, regulates ovarian activity. If overstimulated by excess light, these glands can delay or inhibit ovulation. Louise Lacey, author of *Lunaception,* discovered that light affects the ovulatory cycle via the pineal gland. Too much light, especially at night, overstimulates the pineal gland and causes an imbalance of the hormone melatonin, which in turn overstimulates the hypothalamus and pituitary glands, interrupting the menstrual cycle.

To find out whether or not you are exposed to "too much light," compare your light environment with the cycle of natural light. Women exposed only to natural sunlight and moonlight experience very clear mucus patterns and more regular cycles, with ovulation usually occurring at the full moon and menstruation at the new moon. Pitch-black nights without moonlight are often altered in today's world—"city glow" comes through the bedroom window, and stray light is emitted by clock radios or night lights.

The natural periodicity of light is also distorted by indoor electrical lighting. These forms of light pollution can overstimulate the pineal gland, causing irregular cycles, delayed ovulation, and in some cases, anovulatory (non-egg releasing) cycles.

To prevent light pollution, simply darken the bedroom by placing a blanket over the window and eliminating indoor sources of light. Allow light in only during a few nights in the middle of each cycle (around days fourteen to sixteen, for example). This simulates the natural light cycle and often helps regulate the ovulatory cycle. Fertile mucus patches become shorter and clearer.

Full-Spectrum Light

Another way light can impede fertility (and health) is through imbalanced light rays. Eyeglasses, windows, contacts, and sunglasses filter out 99 percent of ultraviolet light, interfering with the production of melatonin and interrupting the menstrual cycle. Imbalanced light rays affect the body via the eyes. The current fad of totally screening out ultraviolet light may be partly responsible for the increase in infertility, since it appears that balanced light rays are necessary for maintaining fertility.

Ultraviolet light is only a small part of the electro-magnetic spectrum, which includes X-rays, microwaves, infrared rays, gamma rays, and the visible color spectrum. Many of these light rays have been shown to be both healing and harmful, depending on the amount to which one is exposed.

X-rays, for example, can both cure and cause cancer. Radio waves (ultrasound) can detect fetal defects or diseases but may adversely affect the fetus' hearing. Significant increases in leukemia rates have been reported in children living near high-voltage power lines. These and other examples illustrate that an imbalance of electro-magnetic light rays can affect our health. A lack of sufficient ultraviolet light particularly seems to be a culprit in health and fertility problems.

Exposure to full-spectrum light enables the absorption of ultraviolet rays in sufficient and balanced amounts, and glass can counteract this. Factories using full-spectrum lights report increased productivity and lower illness and absentee rates among their workers. To remedy infertility problems, try getting out in natural sunlight, wearing full-spectrum eyeglasses or lenses, spending time under full-spectrum indoor lighting, or using full-spectrum glass for window panes.

Saliva and Other Lubricants

Amylese, an enzyme in saliva, inhibits sperm motility, as do several pharmaceutical lubricating gels. Although these substances do not constitute a major infertility factor, men and women using these lubricants during intercourse may find that it adds one more strike against the possibility of becoming pregnant. Alternative lubricants include egg whites (after checking for egg allergies) or extended foreplay for stimulating increased amounts of vaginal arousal fluid.

Frequency of Intercourse

Engaging in intercourse several days in a row may lower sperm counts and decrease the chances of pregnancy. After ejaculation, thirty to forty hours are needed to build up a new sperm count to peak quantity. Spacing intercourse two to three days apart optimizes the number of sperm available.

Pelvic Alignment

Proper body balance and blood flow to the pelvic area are vital to reproductive health. Imbalanced bloodflow, as evidenced by varicose veins (in testicles and legs), may impair fertility. Applied kinesiology, chiropractic, acupuncture, osteopathy, and other manipulative therapies can provide realignment. Kegel exercises are also helpful for easing any bloodflow restriction caused by tensed pubococcygeus muscles. (Note: It is thought that failure to progress during labor may be caused by pelvic misalignment; imbalanced bloodflow would cause the cervix to dilate unevenly, making it impossible to fully dilate. Having a simple preventative realignment before labor may help prevent this problem.)

Clothing

Ann Landers was right—trashing "tight whites" can increase a man's fertility! Sperm production is optimal when the testicles are not pressed against the body. Pushed against the body in tight pants and underwear, testicles become overheated, resulting in lowered sperm counts and higher numbers of abnormal sperm. Other overheating factors include extended bicycle riding, hot-tubbing, sitting on hard chairs for long periods of time, prolonged hot baths and showers, and working in overheated environments (such as in front of pizza ovens).

It is wise to wear loose clothing and avoid practices that may overheat the testicles. If unable to avoid excess testicular heat on the job, consider the Repro-Med Testicular Hypothermia Device. Worn like a jock-strap, this device contains a reservoir of circulating water which cools the testes.

Drugs

Narcotics, alcohol, tranquilizers, some antidepressants, and antihypertensives may interfere with the ability to ejaculate and thus contribute to retrograde ejaculation (sperm passing into the bladder rather than through the urethra). Alcohol, marijuana, stimulants, antimalarial drugs, nitrofurantoin, methotrexate, tobacco, lithium carbonate, and ulcer medications may lower sperm counts and increase the percentage of abnormal sperm. Tobacco smoking decreases fertility in women, and decongestants and antihistamines can dry up cervical mucus and thus interfere with sperm transport and survival. Marijuana has also been shown to disrupt the ovulatory cycle. To avoid relying on fertility-harming drugs for conditions requiring therapy, use alternative treatments. (For example, fresh cabbage juice effectively improves ulcers.)

Synthetic Hormones

Synthetic hormones are known to cause reproductive abnormalities. Diethylstilbestrol (DES), a synthetic estrogen given to pregnant women between 1941 and 1971, is responsible for reproductive problems in their offspring. Many DES sons have lowered sperm counts; DES daughters often experience intermenstrual bleeding. Both sons and daughters have higher rates of infertility problems than those who were not exposed to DES in utero. To avoid expensive infertility testing, seek care from an experienced DES physician.

Women who discontinue using the contraceptive pill, another synthetic hormone, often experience temporary infertility. Ovulation can be delayed for weeks, months, or in rare cases, a year or two. Mucus charting can document the body's gradual return to normal cycling; detoxification therapies such as fasting or glandular supplementation can hasten the return of fertility.

pH Balance

Douches, creams, spermicides, scented or colored toilet paper, vaginal deodorants, tight nylons or clothing, and scented tampons can throw off the vagina's natural bacteria-yeast balance. The resulting pH imbalance can hamper sperm survival. Antibiotics, notorious for causing yeast infections in the process of killing bacteria, often produce an overgrowth of *Candida* (a yeast-like fungi)—an important factor in some infertility problems.

To optimize vaginal health, use simpler products. Take yogurt and acidophilus to replace bacteria killed by antibiotics. Try yeasticides or dietary measures to counteract yeast overgrowth and rebalance the vaginal environment. In general, it is a good idea for women to wear loose clothing that allows proper air flow to the normally self-cleansing vagina.

Environmental Hazards

The pesticides DBCP, PCB, and EDB can cause sperm abnormalities; lead, aluminum, and other toxic metals can accumulate in the body and alter ovarian or testicular function. Radiation or imbalanced light rays from computer display terminals, television sets, or other sources can harm the ovaries and testicles. After exposure to significant radiation, sperm production may not return for up to two years. According to one physician, if sperm production does not return within four years of radiation exposure, it probably will not return at all.

Environmental hazards are best approached preventatively. Avoid pesticide exposure by eating organically-grown foods. Check water supplies for toxic chemicals and, if necessary, invest in a water purifier to remove toxic metals and chemicals, including chlorine. Also consider a video display terminal (VDT) screen to filter out harmful emissions.

Infections

Mycoplasma, an infectious microorganism, which colonizes on and destroys sperm tails, inhibits sperm motility. One doctor estimates that 40 percent of male infertility problems may be caused by such infections, which can be alleviated with antibiotic therapy.

Herbs

The ingestion of some herbs can interfere with the implantation of a fertilized egg. Blue cohosh, ergot, goldenseal, and pennyroyal all have abortifacient effects. Herbs said to induce ovulation include licorice, unicorn roots, Mexican wild yam, false unicorn root, black cohosh, and elder flowers. Consult with a qualified herbalist for guidance and more information.

Endometriosis

Endometrial cells, normally found only in the uterus, can migrate to other parts of the body and continue to form tissue. The presence of endometrial tissue on the ovaries and fallopian tubes, a condition known as endometriosis, is responsible for approximately 30 to 40 percent of infertility in women. The best way to avoid endometriosis is to prevent situations which can lead to retrograde menstruation (the backing up of menstrual flow through the fallopian tubes). Tampon use may be responsible for some cases of retrograde menstruation and endometriosis.

Stress

Mental, physical, environmental, aural, or visual overstimulation may cause a stress reaction in the body. Stress affects the hypothalamus gland, which regulates appetite, temperature, and emotions. This in turn affects the pituitary gland, which can then delay or prevent ovulation or suppress sperm production. Evaluating stress levels in response to various stimuli is enormously helpful. Meditation, biofeedback, and positive imagery techniques can help counteract the negative effects of stress.

Negativity

Negative thoughts have been shown to produce negative circumstances. Positive thoughts or affirmations create positive results. Affirming positive impressions about fertility and pregnancy may create the desired psychological experience. For example, repeatedly writing a statement such as "I am fertile," or "I am receiving a baby right now" can override negative messages and re-program the unconscious mind to accept the possibility of pregnancy.

Additional Self-Help Tips for Infertility

Short-term vitamin C therapy has been shown to reverse sperm agglutination (clumping) in men. In one study, 500 milligrams of vitamin C every twelve hours yielded positive results within a week. The semen of men with sperm agglutination has been found to be low in vitamin C, zinc, magnesium, calcium, and potassium.

The amino acid L-arginine increases sperm counts and motility. The recommended dosage is four grams per day.

Over-the-counter expectorants (cough syrups) are taken by some to thin cervical mucus that appears "overly thick at ovulation." Biochemically speaking, ovulatory fertile mucus must be very thin and full of channels (for sperm transport); therefore, this treatment seems appropriate only if ovulation is occurring after the fertile mucus stops or when a woman's mucus is "allergic" to the man's sperm. I have seen no documentation of expectorant success and am not convinced that thick mucus at ovulation could actually occur. However, those wishing to consider this option should look for expectorants which contain guaifenesin and avoid those containing ingredients such as codeine.

According to the results of five studies, sperm counts are naturally higher in the winter than in the summer. This may be due to the fewer hours of light available in the winter, or to the cooler weather.

Mumps after puberty can cause testicular damage, as can gonorrhea. The best advice is to avoid these diseases.

Infertile couples can take many steps to evaluate what may be contributing to their infertility problem before going to the doctor. First, it is important to recognize that often *only one small part* of the entire fertility process may be impeded. This helps counteract the overwhelming feeling of being totally infertile or that the body "just isn't working at all." Then, learn to understand your fertility and see how something quite simple—and easily reversible—can affect the ability to conceive a child.

Infertility is not the mysterious and hopeless condition it was once thought to be. There is hope, and there are simple ways to regain fertility. Perhaps the rising incidence of infertility is simply a way for our bodies to let us know that we need to pay more attention to what we do with our bodies and our world.

By *Suzannah Cooper*

For further information,
contact her at P. O. Box 305; Corvallis, OR 97339

SECTION 5

The Second Stairstep: Combining Low-Tech With Medicine

Introduction

When couples are infertile, their first inclination may be to rush to a doctor, but in this section, Ginny Cassidy-Brinn, Carol Downer, and Francie Hornstein ask if difficulty getting pregnant is, in fact, a medical problem. Writing in *Woman-Centered Pregnancy and Birth*, these astute women believe that women are indeed experiencing more difficulty getting pregnant, but they also believe that the problem of fertility is overrated.

Emphasizing procedures that help women pinpoint their fertile times, they explore minor, common surgical procedures that often help, including cryosurgery, laparoscopy, laparotomy, and dilation and curettage (D&C).

When an infertile couple decides to mix low-tech approaches to infertility with low-tech (or high-tech) medicine, they must seek a physician who is knowledgeable about and empathetic with their situation. Dr. Mark Perloe and Linda Gail Christie explore "Finding the Right Doctor" and offer suggestions that will be of immeasurable help to the couple seeking a physician who is not only competent, but who also understands.

New infertility treatments that are done in a doctor's office will have great appeal to many couples. Charles Petit, science writer for the *San Francisco Chronicle*, reports on a new low-cost infertility treatment that requires no hospitalization and takes less than an hour.

Elizabeth Noble, a recognized expert on donor insemination (DI), explores this old but still controversial means of becoming pregnant. Her article describes how she, with her husband's good will, inseminated herself with a friend's sperm.

Ms. Noble's article defines donor insemination and describes this procedure's long history (donor insemination dates back to about 200 B.C.). She also includes the kinds of DI that are used today, the results to be expected, the sex ratio of female versus male children, and the hazards of DI. Ms. Noble also challenges the practice of secrecy associated with DI under the medical model and insists that it can lead to family dysfunction, as it has with adoption. Anonymity keeps a child from knowing her/his genetic heritage, and the use of unknown donor sperm is not as safe as one might hope.

For couples who prefer not to use DI themselves but would invoke the help of a physician, the middle road of openness and cooperation between doctor and patient is essential.

Difficulty Getting Pregnant—A Medical Problem?

Authors of popular articles claim that 18 to 45 percent of couples who want a baby are unable to do so due to infertility. Although we believe that women are experiencing more difficulty getting pregnant due to complications of the Pill and the I.U.D., we believe that the problem of fertility is being overrated. Couples have described years of suffering, of feeling like barren failures. How much of their feelings are due to the medical profession's definition of them as having a medical "condition"? Many people are surprised to learn that only 80 percent of average, healthy women having coitus three or more times a week get pregnant during the first year, and only 65 percent get pregnant during the first six months. It seems impossible to believe so many women could be infertile. We think it takes longer for women to get pregnant than we have been led to believe.

Trying to get pregnant can be difficult and sometimes very discouraging. At what point do you decide that it is time to seek medical help? After one year? Two years? Five years? The answer to this question is individual, but much of what is done by even the most sophisticated infertility specialist can be done just as well by any motivated lay woman, especially if she joins a self-help group. In addition, much of what can't be done by anyone in the privacy of her own home is of dubious value—drugs and surgery that in addition to posing health hazards also my end up actually making it harder for a woman to get pregnant in the long run. If you do decide to seek medical help, a description of the drugs and procedures most commonly done by fertility specialists follows so that you can make informed decisions about your care.

A woman who works with the Feminist Women's Health Centers told us that it took her four years of trying to finally get pregnant. Interestingly, this was two years less than the six years that it took her mother to get pregnant. She said that both she and her mother had kept extensive temperature charts, which didn't seem to help either of them very much. After her mother got pregnant, she quickly gave birth to four more children in less than ten years.

Despite knowing about her mother's experience, the woman told us that she often got very discouraged and thought about going to a physician. But when she and her husband analyzed their situation, they realized that she had actually been out of town for about a fifth of the four years, which meant that she had been gone for almost a year.

She said that it was always tempting to her to put herself under the care of a physician and let him take over and do all the worrying. But whenever she considered seeking medical help, she would go over the alternatives and realize that the bad effects of the drugs and surgery were not something she wanted to risk. Now, looking back, she is glad she decided to avoid medical treatments. She has had two children.

What if she had been one of the unlucky women who get scar tissue that causes blockage of the egg tubes from a diagnostic laparotomy? She only has four or five periods a year. What if she had taken Clomid, a drug that induces ovulation, and happened to stop ovulating altogether after quitting? She thinks that her body probably picked the best time to get pregnant since she was healthier than she had ever been in her life. At that time, she was eating well, taking a lot of vitamin supplements, and running two or three miles a day.

Since multiple factors usually cause infertility, a woman or a couple using a physician or clinic to help the woman get pregnant can expect the process to be an investigative one that can take as long as two years. About one-half of the women who seek medical help eventually get pregnant. However, many of these women might have gotten pregnant anyway without medical help if they had simply kept trying during the months or years they spent attending the fertility clinic.

Detecting Ovulation

All of the methods women use in pinpointing ovulation for the purpose of *not* getting pregnant can also be used to figure out the best time for trying to get pregnant, such as doing vaginal self-examination to become familiar with cervical changes throughout a few cycles, and monitoring the consistency of cervical mucus, and keeping a temperature chart. Some women know exactly when they ovulate each month; they may even feel pain on the right or left side, which lets them know whether the egg was released from the right or left ovary. Many women, however, need to keep track of the signs of ovulation for two or three menstrual cycles before they are able to predict when they will ovulate.

Basal Body Temperature

Constructing a basal body temperature chart, the basis for the rhythm method of birth control, is probably the most commonly used method of fertility awareness. It is based on the fact that the temperature rises slightly with ovulation and stays up until menstruation starts.

Since eating or drinking, smoking, and even a slight amount of activity can affect body temperature, the most accurate way to measure temperature is to take it at the same time every day immediately upon awakening, before even sitting up in bed. One physician reported women taking their temperature within the first few minutes after getting up and still being able to tell when they ovulated. A basal body thermometer, available from most drugstores, makes it easier to read small changes in temperature, but is no more accurate than an everyday fever thermometer. It is not necessary to actually read the temperature or record it on a chart first thing in the morning. The thermometer can be set aside and read later that day. The temperature can be taken from under the tongue or armpit, or in the vagina or rectum, but it is important to take it the same way every time.

Physicians, clinics, and books on natural birth control provide charts on which to record the temperature changes, but a piece of graph paper works fine. These charts show several days of fairly constant temperature after a menstrual period followed by a drop which is then immediately followed the next couple of mornings by a fairly sharp rise of 0.3 to 0.6 degrees. This rise after the drop in temperature is indicative of ovulation. The temperature drops again before menstruation starts.

As the Feminist Self-Insemination Group showed by comparing the charts made up by the real-life women in their group to the classic charts in books, each woman has her own individual pattern. In a review of eleven studies of the menstrual cycle done in five countries, one researcher found that not one woman had a perfectly regular cycle over a significant period of time. Almost no women have a chart that looks exactly like those in books and, at first, it's hard to tell when you ovulate. The Feminist Self-

Insemination Group suggests that, in general, ovulation has occurred when three consecutive temperatures are at least 0.4 degrees Fahrenheit above the previous six days' temperatures. If the temperature rises for less than three days, the woman has probably not ovulated. These brief temperature rises could be caused by factors not related to ovulation, such as illness (even a slight cold), fatigue, lack of sleep, or even electric blankets.

> Since I am a lesbian, and I planned to use artificial insemination, it was important to have an accurate estimate of ovulation in order to maximize the effectiveness of the insemination. I decided to try to pinpoint the time of my ovulation by using the basal body temperature method.
>
> I had read very little about the method, and, in fact, didn't even know what sign would indicate ovulation. I just went ahead and looked for the special basal body temperature thermometer. I finally located one in a larger drugstore. Small drugstores did not carry them. The thermometer had complete instructions and included several blank charts to record my daily temperatures.
>
> It really was a project, requiring that I keep my thermometer next to my bed at all times so I could immediately stick it in my mouth when I woke up. The first two months I had false starts and had to discontinue keeping track. The first month I got a cold and had a slight fever and the second month I got the flu. By the third month I had learned some tricks that helped me get through enough cycles—three, as it turned out—to be able to see that my temperature did create a regular pattern which suggested that I ovulate on my twelfth or sixteenth day.
>
> I broke two basal body temperature thermometers during the first two months of my project. Since they cost five dollars each I decided that from that point on I would just use a regular thermometer, which was cheaper. It worked fine and I never broke my ninety-eight-cent one.

Mucus Detection

More and more women are keeping track of changes in vaginal mucus for birth control or to get pregnant. They find a benefit of this method is that they become more aware of their own bodies and cycles. As long as she makes daily observations, a woman using the mucus detection method can determine fertile days even when ovulation is unpredictable, such as when she has long or irregular cycles, after discontinuing birth control pills, after abortion and childbirth, during lactation, and as menopause begins.

Since the 1930s various researchers have studied the properties of cervical mucus and its effects upon sperm. They placed samples of different cervical mucus on slides, added sperm, and studied it under a microscope. In one type of mucus they saw sperm swimming along parallel streams. In another type of mucus the movement of sperm was chaotic, less vigorous, and stopped sooner. They noted that the first kind of mucus was alkaline and the other was acidic; the first stretched and the other broke apart readily. The alkaline, stretchy mucus appeared around mid-cycle, and the other mucus appeared at other times. Since this alkaline stretchy mucus was present around the time of ovulation they assumed it enhanced fertility and called it fertile mucus.

Within eight to ten hours after the sperm enter the uterus, white blood cells engulf and kill most of them. However, many sperm are harbored in the fertile mucus-secreting cervical glands and are released gradually over a three to five day period. Thus, if fertile mucus is present, sperm entering the vagina up to five days before ovulation can result in pregnancy.

Fertile mucus is alkaline, as is semen, and sperm have been observed to swim more vigorously and live longer in alkaline environments. Nonfertile mucus is acid and sperm have been observed to be immobilized and die sooner in acidic environments.

Some women can detect ovulation simply by observing changes in their mucus secretions, since the changes are dramatic. Others have days when they have difficulty distinguishing fertile mucus from other secretions. Although one kind of mucus is usually dominant, several kinds of mucus are often present. Current research has found that the majority of mucus-producing cells in the cervix are capable of secreting either fertile or nonfertile mucus. Occasionally, a few groups of cells specialize and produce only one kind of mucus, either fertile or nonfertile.

Fertile mucus has several distinct characteristics. Women describe it as slick, slippery, lubricative, transparent, gelatinous, stretchy, stringy, or as having the consistency of raw egg white. It does not easily soak into toilet paper yet may be runny. As it dries, it appears rubbery and yellowish on panties and sometimes even stiffens the crotch. The most marked characteristic of fertile mucus is that it can be stretched.

Women have described nonfertile mucus as milky, like a mixture of flour and water, and sticky or tacky like paste or drying paint. It may be white or yellowish. One of the most important characteristics of nonfertile mucus is that it does not stretch between two points; when stretched it immediately breaks apart.

Following menstruation, women have either no mucus, wet mucus, or sticky, tacky mucus. Then, the mucus becomes slippery and stretchy as ovulation approaches. The stretchiness of the mucus is called (in medical books) *spinnbarkeit*. Sometimes, a woman can stretch this mucus an inch or more without it breaking. The Billings, two Australian researchers, suggest that the last day when fertile mucus is present is generally a woman's most fertile day, at which time she sees the most mucus with the greatest amount of stretchiness.

More than one interval of fertile mucus in a cycle occurs most often in women with cycles longer than twenty-eight days. If the mucus becomes lubricative and stretchy more than once during the same cycle, it could mean that the first episode of fertile mucus was not followed by ovulation.

Some women have mucus so heavy that they see a whitish or yellowish tinge on their panties every day, or mucus so slight that they have to insert their fingers into their vaginas to feel any moisture at all. Mucus ranges from very watery to extremely thick. The amount, color, and consistency of a woman's mucus can stay the same each day or can vary greatly. Regardless of these variations, detection of fertile mucus depends on recognizing when the mucus strings or stretches.

Vaginal Self Examination

Looking directly at her cervix with a speculum, flashlight, and mirror gives a woman a wealth of information about her menstrual cycle. Instead of waiting for the mucus to appear on her panties or toilet paper, she can see it coming out of the opening to the uterus. She can also see cyclical changes in the cervix that are very accurate indications of ovulation.

A woman using a speculum gets precise information even if her mucus is scanty or difficult to classify. When discharge from a vaginal infection makes it difficult to see the mucus, women have found that they can insert the speculum, swab off the discharge on the cervix, and look to see if the os is open and if fertile mucus is coming out of the os.

Most women see that during the days after menstruation the os is relatively closed, and there is little or no mucus coming out. As ovulation approaches, women notice that the os opens and that fertile mucus comes out or appears as a bubble poised at the opening. If a woman touches this mucus with a swab, it can stretch several inches out past the speculum. After ovulation, the os gradually closes and opens again during menstruation.

Once a woman sees her os close after having seen fertile mucus, she can assume that her fertile time is over for that cycle and that she will not be fertile again until after her next menstrual period. Using a speculum in combination with other methods helps a woman precisely identify her fertile time.

Other Signs of Ovulation

Some women see or feel additional signs of ovulation: pain in the region of an ovary (*mittelschmerz*), spotting, or brown or blood-tinged mucus, backache, or feelings similar to pre-menstrual discomfort. One physician reported that women who felt their cervix for fertile mucus often noticed that the position of their cervix shifted higher in the vagina and was harder to reach around the time of ovulation. The elevation of the cervix happens gradually over a four to six day period until ovulation, when it descends again within two to three days.

An additional method of detecting ovulation includes looking under a microscope at slides of cells taken from the vagina with a cotton swab (a vaginal smear) to observe the shape, quality, quantity, and type of cells. This is done to look for an increased rate of cell growth at mid-cycle which would indicate that ovulation had occurred. These smears should be taken daily for one full cycle. A vaginal smear is an imprecise and, at best, indirect method of evaluating ovulation, although we noticed in our own menstrual cycle study that some characteristic changes do occur.

All fertility awareness techniques are time-consuming. They involve not only daily observations but also careful record-keeping. For many women the participation and cooperation of their sex partner is crucial to making the methods practical. Other women use these methods without the knowledge or cooperation of their sex partner or partners.

One self-help woman who used cycle observation as a method of birth control for several months reported:

> When my long-term relationship with my lover became less committed and less predictable, I no longer felt confident in using cycle observation for birth control. I realized that his support, daily participation, and interest had been a vital factor in making the method work.

Maximizing the Chance of Getting Pregnant

Being able to get pregnant, for most women who have not gotten pregnant easily, usually involves maximizing their chances of getting pregnant rather than having a particular condition corrected. Physicians specializing in infertility have found that there is seldom a single reason why it is difficult for a particular woman to get pregnant. There are usually multiple factors. A typical example would be a woman who has irregular periods and doesn't ovulate very often and a man with a sperm count that is on the low side of normal. This situation would significantly cut down the couple's chances of having the sperm meet the egg, but it doesn't make it impossible. This is good news because it means that most women and men can take simple, common sense measures and enhance their fertility without resorting to drugs or surgery.

Timing

It is important for a woman trying to get pregnant to have sperm in her vagina often enough without the man ejaculating too frequently. Heterosexual couples are advised by fertility specialists to have coitus once every forty-eight hours during the woman's fertile time. Based on average sperm counts, this is usually the highest number of ejaculations a man can have without lowering the number of healthy sperm. It is important for the man to avoid ejaculating at all between the scheduled times. This is also relevant for women using donor insemination if they are using the same donor each time. A woman using different donors, on the other hand, can have more frequent inseminations. Some physicians make it a practice to inseminate their clients every day during their fertile time. A woman using different donors can optimize her chances of getting pregnant by getting the donors to abstain from ejaculating for forty-eight hours before donating their semen.

Whether a woman is getting pregnant by coitus or by donor insemination, she has to consciously plan and arrange something that is usually thought of as spontaneous. For heterosexual couples, trying to get pregnant involves having sex on a timetable and may mean having coitus when one or both of the partners is tired or not in the mood. It may also involve restraining from having coitus as frequently as they want to. In the case of privately arranged donor insemination, trying to get pregnant means making complicated arrangements to meet the donor to obtain semen at the right time in the woman's cycle. Many women have reported that the longer it took them to get pregnant, the more difficult it became to convince donors to accommodate busy schedules to provide semen when it was needed. Medically arranged insemination is probably the most convenient way of arranging to get sperm into the vagina, but even these women find themselves driving long distances and rearranging their schedules in order to pick up the semen at the right time and, furthermore, these inseminations are extremely costly—at least 75 to 100 dollars per insemination.

Increasing Sperm Count

Low sperm count is one of the most common causes of difficulty getting pregnant. However, it is still possible for one sperm to reach an egg even if there are very few of them. A common, easily remedied reason for a low sperm count is that the man is ejaculating too frequently.

Sperm live in the scrotal sac in the testicles and are used to being kept at 2.2 degrees centigrade lower than body temperature. The man who wears constricting clothing such as athletic supports or very tight pants for long periods might be pushing the testicles tight enough against his body to raise the temperature of the testicles and kill or damage sperm. Long, hot baths, showers, saunas, or steam baths could also damage some of the sperm.

A sperm count done in a laboratory is a simple, non-invasive way to find out more about possible barriers to the woman's being able to get pregnant. The man is asked to not ejaculate for one or two days before the test. He then ejaculates into a cup, which must be taken to the laboratory within two hours. The technician looks at the sperm under a microscope and sees how many of them there are, how mobile they are, and what percentage of them appear healthy. They also measure the total amount of semen. If the tests indicate there are any problems with the man's sperm, it is a good idea to repeat the test to make sure it is accurate.

A key factor in sperm production is the man's general level of health. A good diet, vigorous exercise, and avoiding harmful health habits such as drinking and smoking might make enough difference in the number or health of the sperm to enable a woman to get pregnant. Some specific vitamins that are often recommended by nutritionists are vitamins A, D, and E. B vitamins, especially pantothenic acid, are sometimes suggested along with the minerals zinc and manganese.

Occasionally, a man with a low sperm count has a varicose vein in the scrotal sac, usually on the left side. In these cases, infertility specialists recommend surgery to tie it off. Surgeons who perform this procedure are not sure how it helps to increase the sperm count. One theory is that the temperature in the testicles becomes too high due to the enlargement of the vein and increased amount of blood it holds. Another theory is that the slow flowing blood in a varicose vein does not allow sufficient oxygen to get to the testicles and allows toxic waste products to accumulate in the area, preventing the sperm from developing optimally.

This surgery involves an abdominal incision, general anesthesia, and hospitalization. Like fertility surgery done on women, it is not always successful, and it seems reasonable to assume that the man runs the risk that rearrangement of the bloodflow to the testicles would end up causing further problems. It is hard to know how frequently this surgery injures the testicles and sperm production since the men who have the surgery already had low sperm counts.

Rarely, a man has no sperm at all in his semen. This is possible due to the tube blockage. A biopsy of both testicles can reveal whether they are producing any sperm at all or whether a tube blockage is keeping sperm which are being produced from being ejaculated.

Illness, especially illnesses in which the man has a high fever for a long time, may lower the sperm count temporarily. Severe stress affects the entire body, including the testicles and sperm production, and could be a factor in a low sperm count for some men.

Infections

An infection of the uterus, tubes, or ovaries can make getting pregnant more difficult. Continuing, chronic inflammation of the cervix, called cervicitis, is thought to interfere with the action of the fertile mucus. The tubes of the endocervical glands which branch deep into the cervix will not be a favorable environment for sperm if they are filled with bacteria and a pus-like discharge. Although a woman with cervicitis can still get pregnant, her chances will improve if the inflammation is cleared up. Cervicitis can be caused by an infection or an irritation, abrasion, or trauma. Women have developed cervicitis from bacterial infections, viral infections, gonorrheal infections, and fungi. Women who use certain birth control methods seem to get cervicitis more often than those who do not. Plus, women who have just given birth can get an infection if the cervix has suffered lacerations during delivery. Scarring on the cervix from giving birth or from tears which sometimes result from the metal instrument used to hold the cervix steady during an abortion can make a woman more prone to cervicitis if irregularities on the cervix provide a place for bacteria to grow.

Self-helpers speculate that many persistent cases of cervicitis can be caused by a chronic infection of the endocervical glands. The tubes of the endocervical glands branch deep into the cervix and can harbor bacteria. When they become infected, an off-white or yellowish discharge comes out of the os. This discharge can burn or irritate any tissue it comes in contact with, including the face of the cervix. These infections are difficult to treat with surface applications. Apparently, even when the signs of illness subside, bacteria remain in the recesses of the glands. When the body's resistance is lowered, the problem flares up again and can possibly spread to the vagina, thus accounting for certain recurring vaginal infections.

There are other cases of cervicitis which have an obvious cause and will probably clear up as soon as the cause is eliminated. We know, for instance, that the trauma of rape can precipitate a flare-up. Additionally, women who use I.U.D.s almost always have a raw patch of red where the string lies on the cervix, and it is not unusual for the string to be covered with pus and mucus, accompanied by runny discharge and blisters, Other women attribute the irritation on their cervixes to vaginal infections which do not respond to treatment.

Self-Help Remedies for Cervicitis

One woman in a self-help group developed a bacterial infection along with gonorrhea. The gonorrhea was successfully treated, but she could not find an adequate remedy for the bacterial infection, which spread into the cervical canal and caused her entire cervix to become red and raw, producing a copious discharge from the os. She described her cervix as looking like "raw meat." She used a remedy suggested by other members of her self-help group with great success. For two weeks she daubed vitamin E oil on her cervix with a cotton swab, and it healed perfectly.

Some women have noticed that the redness of their cervixes has cleared up without any treatment at all. Others have successfully used home remedieswhich appear to work very well for these minor irritations.

One woman had a friend apply honey to her cervix with a cotton swab and found that it cleared up her minor irritation.

Another woman had satisfactory results when she had a friend apply the juice from an aloe vera plant (a spiny cactus that contains a juice that has long been used for healing and is a main ingredient in many first aid creams) to the reddened area on her cervix.

In situations where coitus causes irritation of the cervix, abstinence or changes in positions might alleviate the symptoms.

Many times, a vaginal infection is the underlying cause of cervicitis, so, treating either with any of these home remedies can, in the process, clear up the other.

It is even possible that some of the irritations that we treat with home remedies would have cleared up on their own without the user of self-help remedies, but this in no way suggests that these remedies are not effective and should not be tried for alleviating discomfort. Further study and research on the use of home remedies for curing cervicitis and other vaginal ailments is being done in ongoing self-help groups.

Cauterization of the Cervix

If the inflammation and accompanying discharge or bleeding does not cease with home remedies, or if it is causing pain or has not cleared up before it is time for a regular examination, a woman can request medication.

Drugs that are usually prescribed are antibiotics such as tetracycline or an antibacterial cream such as AVC cream, a sulfa-based drug. One of these treatments usually takes care of the inflammation. If not, most physicians will recommend cauterization, which freezes the top layer of cells from the cervix with liquid nitrogen (cryosurgery) or by burning the cervix with a hot electrocautery instrument so that old cells will die and be sloughed off and new, healthy cells can grow.

Women in self-help groups have repeatedly related stories of having their cervixes cauterized. It is clear to the women's health movement, after thousands of women have done routine self-exams, that physicians cauterize cervixes unnecessarily. It has been customary for physicians to cauterize every red cervix they see. It was not until very recently that medical students were taught that what had been called cervicitis or an "eroded cervix" is actually a cervix with a visible squamo-columnar junction, or a cyclical coloration of the cervix. Despite the medical profession's belated acknowledgment of something that self-help groups saw immediately, too many women continue to be subjected to the discomfort and expense of repeated, unnecessary, and traumatic cauterization of their healthy cervixes.

One woman who had her cervix cauterized numerous times eventually needed surgery to enlarge her cervical canal because scar tissue blocked the menstrual flow. In another instance, a physician was asked by a health worker who was assisting why he had cauterized a woman's cervix. His reply was, "So it will look pretty for the next doctor she sees."

By doing self-examination, we can know how long a redness has been there, if it is the squamo-columnar junction and is normal for us, or if there has been some reason for irritation such as trauma or infection. Many women are now resisting when their physicians tell them they need cauterization. A woman might want to go home and periodically examine her cervix before deciding to have it cauterized. With all the information she has about the squamo-columnar junction, reasons for cervicitis, knowledge of home remedies, and particularly with the ability to do routine self-examination, the woman knows that cauterization needs to be done only to correct painful or persistent conditions.

In spite of its overuse, cauterization can be an effective treatment. A good example of this is one self-helper who had cervicitis caused by a severe infection in the endocervical glands. It persisted for over a year, causing a constant, heavy discharge. After trying one home remedy after another and every conventional cure for vaginal infections, including douches, she chose to have cryosurgery. Both the infection and the discharge cleared up immediately, and she has not been bothered by it since.

Cryosurgery

Cryosurgery is considered to be the most effective method of cauterizing the cervix. (It is also sometimes used to remove genital warts.) In this procedure, a cautery tip is connected to a canister of liquid nitrogen, which is changed into gas, freezing the tissues of the cervix. As the cervical cells thaw, they absorb moisture and expand, causing the cell walls to burst, and allowing water from the cells to escape. Dehydration and death of these cells results.

Usually, the freezing is done by holding a cautery tip against the cervix for two or three minutes. This can be repeated after a few minutes' rest. The cryosurgery actually causes an ice ball up to one-fourth of an inch deep to form on the face of the cervix. Gradually, the ice melts and the water and dead cells are sloughed off and flow out of the vagina. This results in a heavy, watery discharge that can last for several days to a few weeks. During this time, a sanitary napkin (not a tampon) needs to be worn.

Women have reported entirely different reactions to freezing, from feeling nothing to feeling severe pain. One woman told us that her physician left the room after freezing her cervix. She remained on the examination table for some time with the metal speculum still inserted. The cryosurgery had frozen the metal speculum to her flesh, and it had to be warmed before it could be removed. This additional procedure was extremely painful, as well as unnecessary.

The discharge after cryosurgery can be very bothersome. It is usually suggested that nothing be introduced into the vagina for three weeks after the procedure to protect the newly exposed cells from infection. It takes about eight weeks for the cervix to be totally healed.

Generally, cauterization with cryosurgery seems to be effective in replacing inflamed cells with healthy ones. However, if the source of the inflammation remains or recurs, these newly exposed cells can then become reinfected. It is important, therefore, to determine the source of the infection and to treat it. Repeated cauterization by any method can cause scarring of the cervix, as well as of the cervical canal and can, among other things, interfere with the flow of menstrual blood.

Cryosurgery is a simple outpatient procedure but is fairly expensive, costing between fifty and seventy-five dollars. Some physicians charge considerably more.

Pelvic Inflammatory Disease

Pelvic inflammatory disease (PID) is a general infection of the uterus, endometritis; the egg tubes, salpingitis; or the ovaries, ovarian abscess. Infection of any one or a combination of those is called PID. Probably the most common cause is untreated gonorrhea, but other causes can be complications from I.U.D.s, surgery, childbirth, or abortions.

A number of women who have had PID are left with long-term problems. Some are bothered by recurrent pelvic infections. Others have a greater risk of having tubal pregnancies and, of course, infertility is a possible problem if the scarring blocks both egg tubes or interferes with implantation of a fertilized egg.

It is common for gonorrhea to progress to PID, since women usually do not have many obvious signs and do not seek treatment until they have signs of PID. In PID caused by gonorrhea infections, the bacteria usually enter through the vagina and cervix. If the infection is untreated, the bacteria slowly migrate up into the uterus. Uterine infections caused by gonorrhea are not too serious in most cases; however, if the infection reaches the egg tubes, it usually causes inflammation which can lead to scarring, blocking of the egg tubes, and infertility. By the time the infection reaches the tubes, a woman usually notices pain in the pelvic region, which appears most often around the time of menstruation.

It is easy to see how the constant irritation of the lining of the uterus by a foreign object such as an I.U.D. could contribute to PID. It is not surprising that this inflammation does not always clear up immediately and that some women have a difficult time getting pregnant after having an I.U.D. removed. As with any pelvic infection, if there is scar tissue the difficulty may be permanent.

A woman might suspect that she had PID if she has pain in the lower part of her abdomen, accompanied by a fever, nausea or vomiting, or a foul-smelling vaginal discharge, which she can see coming directly out of the os. Painful coitus or unusually painful menstrual periods are also signs of PID. If she thinks she may have been exposed to gonorrhea or if she has any of these signs after surgery on her reproductive organs, childbirth, or abortion, the possibility of PID should be considered. Early detection and treatment of PID gives a woman a better chance of becoming pregnant easily when she wants to. Dr. Bernard Rosenfeld, who gained national attention in 1974 for his courageous efforts to expose sterilization abuses at large, inner-city hospitals, studied PID extensively and concluded that by the time a woman starts to have pelvic pain, there is a strong possibility that she has already had scarring.

One way of confirming that a woman has PID is to take a sample of the secretions coming out of the os and send them to a laboratory to be cultured. The results will show the type of infection and which antibiotics would be successful in killing it. A negative culture does not mean that a woman has no pelvic infection, and sometimes the condition is difficult to diagnose. A pelvic examination is usually very painful for a woman who has PID because it hurts to have the uterus, tubes, or ovaries moved if they are inflamed. Although this is one way to diagnose the condition, there are differing opinions of the advisability of a pelvic examination for a woman with suspected PID, since the manipulation of the organs can cause further irritation. It is best, if an examination is done that it be as gentle as possible.

Because inflammation can lead to scar tissue, which has a long-lasting effect on fertility, physicians are eager to do whatever they can to get rid of pelvic infection immediately. They invariably prescribe oral antibiotics. If the woman is unable to take antibiotics due to nausea and vomiting, or if the physician believes that her infection is severe, she might be hospitalized to receive large doses of intravenously administered antibiotics. Another treatment that might be suggested, especially after surgery, is for the uterus and tubes to be washed with a liquid solution of antibiotics and cortisone. The purpose of the antibiotics is to kill bacteria and the purpose of the cortisone is to prevent inflammation. Antibiotics, especially when given intravenously, are powerful drugs with a wide range of undesirable effects from indigestion and diarrhea to kidney failure. Cortisone is also a dangerous hormone-like drug, which is usually made by the adrenal gland. When a woman takes any hormone-like drug, the gland that usually makes the hormone slows or shuts down. In the case of the adrenal gland and cortisone, the body's natural response to any inflammation is inhibited. Every cell in the body is affected.

Despite these dangers, many women choose to use the drugs because they are justifiably concerned about the very real effects of pelvic infection on their future fertility, as well as the severe pain that sometimes results from recurring PID. It is unfortunate that physicians do not usually give women the information about the dangers of these drugs and let them make their own decisions.

Once a woman has had PID, she may find that it recurs throughout her life. Women in this situation have explored alternatives to the traditional antibiotic treatment. One participant in a self-help clinic who had a chronic infection resulting from an I.U.D. complication was able to keep it under control by preventing subsequent flare-ups with home remedies.

Sometimes, women are given the erroneous impression by their physicians that the fact that they have PID means that they can never get pregnant. This is untrue as many women who have had both wanted and unwanted pregnancies after having had PID can testify. In addition to self-help remedies such as vitamin C and herbs, increasing a woman's overall health by a good diet and regular exercise gives her a better chance of getting pregnant. Some women have had the scar tissue removed by surgery, although this is not always successful. Other women have gotten pregnant without trying at all.

In the process of healing itself of damage caused by an I.U.D., a pelvic infection such as gonorrhea, or abdominal surgery, the body often forms scar tissue. This scar tissue can block, or kink the egg tubes or make it difficult for a fertilized egg to implant in the wall of the uterus. When two inflamed surfaces are stuck together, the resulting adhesions can obstruct the passage or implantation of the egg or the sperm.

There are many reports in medical literature of women getting pregnant after surgery who were previously unable to do so. These reports give hope to women who have had an extremely difficult time getting pregnant. Unfortunately, surgeons rarely discuss the unsuccessful cases where women were unable to get pregnant even after surgery and the even more sobering fact that any abdominal surgery, including all types of infertility surgery, can cause infertility. So, a woman who has infertility surgery could end up having an even harder time getting pregnant as a result of the surgery.

Laparoscopy

In an attempt to avoid extensive surgery, many physicians suggest first doing a laparoscopy. The incisions required are much smaller than the incisions for traditional abdominal surgery. If the problem can be taken care of by tiny instruments, the amount of cutting of tissue can be considerably lessened by laparoscopy. However, laparoscopy is being overused.

Sometimes physicians use it merely to satisfy their curiosity, and the additional information provided by the laparoscopy, although interesting, is actually unnecessary.

If tubes are blocked or kinked by scar tissue, fertility specialists recommend surgery to try to repair the damage. The same operation is done for women who want to reverse a tubal ligation. The surgeon cuts out the blocked part of the tube and sews the remaining pieces together or sews the remaining part of the tube to the uterus. If the tube is kinked because of surrounding scar tissue, the surgeon will attempt to remove the scar tissue to free the tube. Removing most of the tube, although it might remove a blockage, could also add another factor making a successful pregnancy more difficult by shortening the amount of time the egg spends in the tube. If the egg is pushed into the uterus before it has time to develop, it might not be mature enough to successfully implant itself in the uterus.

The fimbria, which are the finger-like projections on the end of the egg tubes near the ovary, play an active role in ovulation by wrapping themselves around the ovary and pushing the egg into the egg tube. If they are stuck together or stuck to the ovary, the surgeon will attempt to separate them.

For over a century, people have tried to look inside the body with arrangements of tubes and lights. The major problem was getting the light inside the body without cooking the tissues. The laparoscope is a tube that brings light from the viewer's end through glass fibers to the other end, where tissues can be seen without being heated.

When laparoscopy is done under a local anesthetic, informational counseling is desirable before, during, and after the procedure, because the woman's active cooperation is necessary. If a woman is having a laparoscopy under a local anesthetic, she is often given an opium-like drug and a muscle relaxant (Demerol and Valium) before the procedure. These drugs relax most women, but can cause others to feel panicky or helpless.

The woman's abdomen and some of her pubic mound is usually shaved. Some physicians insert a catheter through the urethra and her bladder is emptied of urine. The woman will be lying on her back on a slant, her head lower than her feet, so that gravity will draw the abdominal organs away from the uterus and tubes. A speculum is inserted and a small suction cup with a handle that sticks out of the vagina is attached to the cervix. This enables the surgeon to move the uterus so it can be seen from all sides through the laparoscope.

A hollow needle is inserted near the navel and about three to four quarts of carbon dioxide are put into the abdomen to lift the abdominal wall away from the organs. The abdomen will dome. Since the gas in the abdomen puts pressure on the diaphragm, a woman must make a conscious effort to breathe. If she is having the procedure done with a local anesthetic, a counselor can remind her to keep breathing. If the woman is having a general anesthetic, breathing will be regulated mechanically.

A small incision, one-eighth to one-half inch, is made in the navel and a pointed metal tube about one-half inch in diameter, called a trocar, is inserted, which pokes and cuts through the layers of fat and muscle. The laparoscope is inserted through the tube. Through the laparoscope, the surgeon sees the organs in the abdominal cavity.

If the surgeon sees evidence of extensive scar tissue and adhesions or any other condition that makes laparoscopic surgery difficult or dangerous, this route has to be abandoned and a laparotomy done instead.

If the surgeon is going to do anything more than look at the organs, a second incision is made near the pubic hairline. Tiny instruments are inserted and manipulated from outside the woman's body while the surgeon observes through the laparoscope.

The introduction of gas into the abdominal cavity can cause a variety of problems. A woman might feel soreness, even extreme discomfort, in her shoulders. The soreness can be avoided if she lies down and does not lift her head for an hour after the procedure. As the body absorbs the gas, the sensations will gradually lessen and disappear.

By mistake, the gas may have been injected into layers of tissue and it can travel under the skin from the groin to the neck. The medical profession considers this to be a minor complication since the tissues and blood absorb the gas and then it is exhaled through the lungs. The trocar tube has a sharp pointed end, and can cut or perforate abdominal organs. If perforation occurs, a larger abdominal incision would be made to repair the perforation.

Women who have had a local anesthetic generally feel well enough to get dressed and leave about an hour or so after laparoscopy. Generally, there is no internal pain, but there can be some soreness where the incisions were made that can last as long as a week. After a general anesthetic, many women feel drained and weak, and it takes several days to several weeks before they have their usual energy.

Laparotomy

Laparotomy is a term used to describe any surgery done with an abdominal incision. This includes abdominal hysterectomy, surgery on fibroids of the uterus or myomectomy, ovarian or egg tube surgery, or bladder surgery. At one time, most incisions were made vertically on the abdomen from anywhere between the navel to the pubic hairline. This vertical incision gives a wider field of view to the surgeon, an everlasting scar to the woman, and can weaken the abdominal wall. Today more horizontal incisions are being done. These are usually made right at the pubic hairline and have been humorously called bikini incisions by surgeons who assume that the only reason a woman would not want a large scar would be so she could wear a bikini. Though it is more difficult for the surgeon to maneuver through this incision, the results are generally superior to the vertical incision, because the cut is made in the same direction as the connective muscle tissue, and then the muscles can be gently pulled to each side. Recovery is faster and less painful. There is also less tension on the incision as it heals because a woman can regulate how straight she stands, and the scarring is generally less obvious when covered by pubic hair.

Recovery from laparotomy takes time and is usually very painful during the three to five days following surgery. Complete overall recovery time is at least three to six weeks and can be longer. Since laparotomy is done with general anesthetic, there can be after-effects such as gas, muscle pain, and fatigue, as well as after-effects from the operation.

Dilation and Curettage (D&C)

Dilation and curettage (D&C) involves dilating or stretching the opening of the uterus with progressively larger smooth metal rods called dilators and then scraping the wall of the uterus with a razor-sharp spoon shaped instrument called a curette. It is the most common gynecological operation. In general, if anything out of the physician's definition of normal happens, a woman can expect a D&C. Sometimes D&C is also done just to be sure that there is nothing out of the ordinary, just to be sure that nothing is wrong.

D&C is often suggested to remove fibroids or polyps for women having difficulty getting pregnant. It is theorized that these benign growths in the lining of the uterus interfere with the fertilized egg being able to implant. This may be true; however, there are risks to a D&C that could make it more difficult for a woman to get pregnant. If her infertility is the result of scanty uterine lining, D&C removes what lining there is and succeeds only in perpetuating the condition, called Ascherman's Syndrome. Uterine adhesions, another cause of infertility, are generally caused by irritation or infection of the uterine lining as might be caused by an I.U.D. Scraping with a metal curette to remove adhesions will undoubtedly irritate the lining causing more adhesions.

We believe D&C is overused and often unnecessary. Vacuum aspiration is a less traumatic technique for abortion and has fewer complications than D&C. The amount of cervical dilation needed is smaller and the procedure can be done under local rather than general anesthetic. If a physician suggests doing a D&C in order to obtain a sample of the uterine lining to determine if the woman is ovulating (endometrial biopsy), this can undoubtedly be done less traumatically and less painfully by using a small, flexible plastic cannula, just as is used in vacuum aspiration abortion. The vacuum aspiration procedure, which is not a surgery, involves no cutting or scraping. A thin plastic tube is inserted through the cervical opening and the contents of the uterus are gently suctioned out.

Exercise and Fertility

Since the whole body is involved in the hormonal changes that make it possible for a man to produce healthy sperm and for a woman to get pregnant, a woman can increase her chances of pregnancy if both she and the prospective father do whatever they can to become as healthy as possible. Regular, strenuous exercise is a major contributor to health, and it makes sense that a woman who is trying to get pregnant would include it as part of her health program.

Women have questioned whether they should exercise if they are having difficulty getting pregnant because of the fact that some women athletes found that they either did not menstruate at all or menstruated very infrequently. On the other hand, many women have said that they were unable to get pregnant until after they began a vigorous exercise program. The women who reported they stopped having periods while exercising were serious athletes exercising many hours a day, whereas the women who reported that exercise helped them get pregnant had been relatively inactive before beginning exercise programs. The athletes found that they were able to get their regular periods back by decreasing the amount of exercise; it was not necessary for them to stop exercising altogether.

Presently, there is actually very little known about the fertility of women athletes. Dr. Joan Ullyot, the author of two excellent books for women runners, speculates that lack of menstruation in an extremely active woman may be a healthy adaptation of the body to there being less than an optimal amount of body fat to support a pregnancy. She points out that the serious, competitive athletes who have this condition often have less than 13 percent body fat, whereas the typical American woman who leads a sedentary life has at least 30 percent body fat. She theorizes that regular menstruation is a phenomenon that has arisen within the past 10,000 years and points out that it would be very inconvenient for nomadic women to be pregnant or nursing small babies for a large part of their lives. She suggests that regular menstruation can only flourish in a "settled and inactive society which can afford to have its women effectively immobilized much of the time." She suggests that an athlete who wishes to become pregnant and hasn't had a period for months or years first discontinue all birth control measures for a year or more. If she still does not become pregnant, she suggests increasing fat percentage by cutting down on exercise to a level that is easy and eating adequately.

The medical treatment for a woman who is not ovulating or who does not have fertile mucus is often hormone-like drugs. Fertility drugs were developed at the same time the birth control pill was developed, and like the birth control pill, the safety of these drugs is questionable and their effectiveness is overrated. One very serious consideration for women taking fertility drugs is that they are not safe to take during pregnancy. Women taking them have had babies with many different types of birth defects. Although it has not been proven that all of these birth defects were actually caused by the fertility drugs, physicians are cautioned by the companies that manufacture them to be very careful about determining if a woman is pregnant before giving the drugs. This is difficult, since it is impossible to know a woman is pregnant in the first few days after conception.

The twenty years that the fertility drugs have been in use is not long enough for anyone to feel confident that all of the serious effects have been documented. All hormone-like drugs affect every part of the body. And, like women who take the birth control pill or estrogen replacement therapy, women who take these drugs are part of an experiment. Years from now, after millions of women have taken fertility drugs, life threatening effects may finally begin to be documented as they have been with the birth control pill.

Experiences of women who have taken the birth control pill or estrogen replacement therapy have shown us that if a hormone or hormone-like drug is taken, the body stops making the hormone on its own, and the glands that make the hormone shrink much like a leg muscle shrinks if the leg is in a cast. Some women do not ovulate for many months after stopping taking the birth control pill. A few women are permanently affected and never ovulate again. We suspect that fertility drugs such as Clomid and Pergonal may in the future be found to have similar effects. Women who only ovulate infrequently might find that after taking these drugs they do not ovulate at all.

Pergonal (menotropins) is a drug containing follicle stimulating hormone (FSH) and luteinizing hormone (LH), which are involved in the development of the egg. This drug, extracted from women's urine, is injected every day for nine to twelve days. Women who have taken Pergonal or similar drugs have had babies with birth defects; however, the manufacturer claims that these birth defects were probably not related to the drug. Since most of the research that has been done on fertility drugs has been financed by the drug companies, it is very hard for a woman considering taking them to evaluate the risks. Women who took Pergonal are even more likely than women who took Clomid to have multiple births. Twenty percent of the pregnancies following treatment with Perganol and similar drugs have resulted in multiple births.

Clomid (clomiphene citrate) is the most well-known and most commonly used of the fertility drugs. It is a hormone-like drug that is thought to encourage the pituitary gland to make more follicle stimulating hormone (FSH), which then causes the egg to develop. Actually, no one knows for sure how the drug works. They do know that women who take it have a higher than average chance of having a multiple pregnancy (7.9 percent of all pregnancies). Since the drug began to be used in the early sixties, some of the bad effects that have been documented include blurred vision and other visual disturbances, abdominal pain, nausea and vomiting, enlargement of the ovaries, headache, dizziness, insomnia, fatigue, depression, hair falling out, weight gain or loss, and jaundice.

If a woman still does not seem to be ovulating after taking fertility drugs, her physician may suggest a laparoscopy to see if she has what is called polycystic ovaries. The ovaries of women who have this condition have many mature eggs, none of which actually break out of the ovary. Sometimes the ovary is enlarged, and often the ovaries are covered by a tough membrane.

Under a general anesthetic with a laparotomy, the woman will have a wedge of tissue removed from each ovary. Although they don't know how it works, surgeons believe that this operation substantially increases a woman's chances of getting pregnant, especially immediately after the operation is performed. As with all fertility surgery, there is the chance that this surgery could cause new scar tissue to form, blocking the egg tubes.

Incompatibility Between Mucus and Sperm

Women who are trying to get pregnant can gather a lot of information simply by charting the changes in their vaginal mucus to see if they regularly have mucus with the stretchy characteristics of fertile mucus. But if a woman wants more information about the effectiveness of her fertile mucus in keeping sperm alive and in transporting it to the egg, it is necessary to take a post-coital test.

A post-coital test is done by taking a small sample of the mucus out of the woman's vagina during the woman's fertile time several hours after coitus or insemination. Sperm can be easily seen under a microscope. If they are still active, the fertile mucus is effectively keeping them alive and helping them to get to the egg. If the sperm are immobile or moving slowly, it is possible that the woman has not calculated her fertile time accurately. Or it could be that she is not ovulating. Another possibility is that a vaginal or cervical infection is interfering with the fertility of the mucus.

There is an extremely rare condition in which a woman has antibodies to sperm. In these cases, the post-coital test will show sperm that are extremely sluggish or immobile. In some of these cases, if the woman's fertile mucus is combined with a different man's sperm, these new sperm will be kept alive and mobile in the woman's fertile mucus, and these women are thought to have antibodies to only one particular man's sperm. Physicians suggest abstaining from contact with sperm for a few months so that the woman's body will stop making antibodies. If a couple has coitus during the period of abstention, the man can use a condom. Blood tests can confirm whether the woman actually has antibodies.

If they are unable to figure out or correct the incompatibility between sperm and mucus, fertility specialists sometimes suggest using insemination with the usual semen. Depositing the semen right at the entrance to the uterus gives the sperm a better chance to reach the egg without the help of the fertile mucus.

By *Ginny Cassidy Brinn, Francie Hornstein, and Carol Downer*

Finding the Right Doctor

Shelley looked toward me. "Dr. Perloe, how can couples find out which doctor to go to?"

"There are a number of alternatives. RESOLVE's list of physicians is an excellent beginning." I paused. "However, one thing that concerns me greatly is the thinking that says that only a fertility specialist can treat fertility problems. That simply is not true."

"But I wasted over a year going to my family doctor before I realized he was just bouncing from one thing to another," Shelley said.

"I know that can happen. But even a fertility specialist may use hit-or-miss procedures. You see, there is nothing to prevent any doctor from hanging up a shingle that says 'fertility specialist.'"

"I didn't know that," Debbie said.

"First consult with your family physician or obstetrician-gynecologist. She or he knows your medical history better than anyone. If your problem requires specialized knowledge, ask your doctor to refer you to a specialist.

"Read everything you can about fertility problems and fertility treatment. Talk to RESOLVE members and other infertile couples about their experiences and compare what's happening to you with what you learn. Talk to your doctor. Discuss your treatment plan and ask lots of questions. If it seems to you that your doctor does not have a plan, is not using 'accepted' procedures, or resents answering your questions, you may want to seek a second opinion."

"What if you don't have a doctor?" a woman across the room asked.

"Get a list of names in your area from the American Fertility Society or your local county medical society. Call or write fertility clinics for additional information. Talk to family and friends, too. Perhaps they know someone who's seeing a doctor for fertility treatment. With one in six couples in the United States seeking treatment for fertility problems, help can't be too far away. The best insurance you can have is being prepared—by reading, attending workshops, and joining support groups."

In the following, I will tell you how to find a physician, what types of physicians or clinics to look for, and how to spot the "poor treatment" danger signs.

Consult Your Current Physician

I encourage you to consult your family practice physician or obstetrician-gynecologist first. Since you've already developed a rapport, it will be easier for you to share personal and intimate facts about your sexual history and habits. Both of these physicians are trained to analyze the results from a semen analysis, blood tests, and X-rays, and they know how to administer fertility treatment to both men and women. The following is a more detailed breakdown of different medical specialties.

Doctors Who Treat Fertility Problems

General Practitioner, Family Physician, Internal Medicine Specialist

Family physicians can assess your general health and investigate the potential effects of medical history, environment, and medications on your fertility. These physicians can determine if a woman is ovulating and if a man's semen is functional. Many common fertility problems may be resolved at this initial level—for example, using a basal body temperature chart to time coitus, ovulation induction, and counseling on the discontinuance of sperm-killing douches and lubricants. If your fertility problem is such that it demands it, your physician should refer you to a specialist. Since your records and test results will be provided to the specialist, you won't have wasted your money by seeing your family doctor first.

Obstetrician-Gynecologist

This physician specializes in the study and treatment of women's diseases, especially of the genitourinary and rectal tracts. In addition, he or she is concerned with the care and treatment of women during pregnancy and childbirth. Most OB-GYNs, as they are commonly called, also perform surgery. However, depending on their skills, they may or may not be able to perform microsurgery on your fallopian tubes, which is required in about 10 percent of fertility patients. Most OB-GYNs can perform a diagnostic laparoscopy, but if they can't do microsurgery, the laparoscopy may have to be repeated by the microsurgeon so he or she can plan your corrective surgery. OB-GYNs have access to all of the fertility diagnostic tests available, including the semen analysis. The OB-GYN should be able to treat anovulation and to perform artificial insemination.

Reproductive Endocrinology and Fertility Specialist

This is an American Board of Obstetrics and Gynecology certified subspecialty for OB-GYNs who receive extra training in endocrinology (the study of hormones) and infertility. Generally these physicians are affiliated with fertility research programs at universities, infertility clinics, or in vitro centers. They have the most up-to-date information on fertility and are skilled in microsurgery techniques.

Urologist

This physician specializes in the male genitourinary tract. The urologist can perform a semen analysis and can examine a man for a varicocele, endocrine problems, genetic defects, or other physical abnormalities that may cause fertility problems. In addition, the urologist can perform a testicular biopsy, surgery for varicocele repair, and vasectomy reversal.

Andrologist

This physician-scientist performs laboratory evaluations of male fertility. The andrologist need not be a medical doctor and may hold a Ph.D. degree in any number of technical areas, including microbiology, biochemistry, or andrology. Many andrologists are affiliated with fertility treatment centers and play a key role in performing in vitro fertilization.

Accepting Your Physician's Referral

If you trust your doctor, you'll be inclined to trust the quality of the referral. Referral from another physician is one of the quickest and best ways to find a doctor.

Starting Your Search from Scratch

If you're faced with finding a new physician on your own, you may want to utilize some of these resources:

1. *RESOLVE, Inc.* Contact your local RESOLVE, Inc. chapter or national RESOLVE, Inc. for a referral.

2. *The American Fertility Society and local county medical society.* As noted, these organizations can provide you with a list of physicians who have expressed an interest in fertility treatment. Although membership in these organizations doesn't certify fertility treatment competency, this may be a good list to work from.

3. *Fertility clinics.* A number of fertility clinics exist across the country. Some of them are for-profit clinics; others are nonprofit research organizations, usually associated with universities. Many of these clinics can perform your fertility workup. If not, they can provide you with a list of the physicians whom they work with in your community.

Should You Go to a Specialist?

Through your reading and search for information, you may have noticed that many sources recommend you avoid your family physician and obstetrician-gynecologist and go directly to a fertility specialist. I have heard couples say, "If you go to the in vitro clinic for your workup, you're getting the best." While it is certainly true that you can receive very good care through these facilities, the erroneous conclusion drawn by some couples is: "If you don't go to the in vitro center, you're settling for second best." Or even worse: "If the in vitro center can't help you, that's the final word."

You may also have heard that you can identify a fertility specialist by the fact that he or she "specializes" in fertility and *doesn't deliver babies*—the logic apparently being that if doctors are busy delivering babies, they're too busy to know enough about fertility to practice it. I don't believe this is an adequate description, however, of a physician who is qualified to treat your fertility problem. So for a number of reasons, which I'll share with you, I disagree with this generalized recommendation for fertility specialists.

Any physician can be listed as a fertility specialist. There is no regulation, licensing, or certification required for advertising this specialty. Before you make your first appointment, however, you can inquire if the physician is *board-certified* in the reproductive endocrinology and infertility subspecialty. To become board-certified, the physician must meet educational requirements and pass written tests.

Membership in the American Fertility Society is available to any physician showing an interest in the specialty. While membership in this organization does not guarantee a known standard of technical competence, it does demonstrate the physician's interest in fertility treatment (a definite plus).

Specialists may charge more for the same services. An article in *Money* magazine stated that fertility specialists may charge up to five times more than nonspecialists. This may be overstated, but before you settle on the physician you want, ask about the charges for common tests and procedures. You may find that you'll pay twenty to twenty-five dollars more for a semen analysis from a specialist, even though the same medical laboratory provides these services to all of the doctors in your community. Do a little price comparison first and remember that the lowest- or highest-priced doctor is not necessarily the worst or best.

The Private Physician vs. the Fertility Clinic

Another question that arises is whether to consult with a private physician or go to a large fertility clinic. A private physician can treat most fertility problems. The additional skills and expertise provided by in vitro centers and large fertility clinics are needed only for about 10 percent of fertility problems. I have some additional ideas on this matter that I'd like to share with you:

For-profit fertility clinics and in vitro centers are not certified and their reported results aren't validated. Fertility treatment has become a big moneymaking business. It's little wonder that the clinic's interest in attracting customers influences the way in which they may report their pregnancy success rates. For example, a clinic may report that 25 percent of their patients get pregnant within three cycles. So you may assume that you have a one in four chance of pregnancy if you go to them. These could look like pretty good odds to some couples. However, the clinic's statistics do not show that they eliminate more than half of the applicants before attempting any in vitro procedures. So in actual fact only 25 percent of the remaining half of their patients (or really 12.5 percent of *all* their patients) actually succeed. Don't get me wrong—many of these clinics are quite reputable and do show impressive results. Just try to be objective when you read or hear about their services and success rates.

Research-oriented clinics may perform unnecessary tests and procedures to meet research criteria and to pay their expenses. In order to conduct scientifically sound fertility research, medical professionals must have similar information about each couple. Thus, this kind of clinic may perform expensive tests not only on patients who warrant them but also on those who do not need them. In this way the researchers can compare their results between "abnormal" and "normal" populations. Consequently the research clinic may not tailor your workup to your unique set of problems. Money charged for these "extra" tests also helps pay the bills for expensive laboratory and research capabilities, which may not be needed for your basic diagnostic workup. Before signing up with a research clinic, find out what diagnostic procedures they recommend and how much they charge. If this information doesn't correlate with what you've learned about fertility treatment, you may wish to get a second opinion.

Larger clinics may contribute to your feeling of isolation and anonymity. Often couples who have gone to large clinics complain that they didn't receive much of the physician's personal time; no one in the clinic knew them by sight; and a different resident physician saw them at each visit. Also, many people who travel considerable distances to these clinics don't feel comfortable expressing their concerns: they feel isolated and dissatisfied. One patient said, "I feel like I'm being herded like cattle." If that's the way you feel, you probably are not getting the personal attention you need, and the clinic you're going to may be too large. I must say, however, that a number of large clinics provide services that many smaller organizations cannot: educational videotapes, nurse practitioners to answer questions, on-site X-ray and testing laboratories, and counseling and support groups—all of which can be of great value.

For-profit fertility clinics tend to charge more for basic diagnostic workups and treatments than do family practitioners and obstetrician-gynecologists. I find that people who go to fertility and in vitro clinics for standard workups and treatment tend to pay *50 to 100 percent more* than those going to private practitioners. These charges result in part from the higher overhead these clinics incur for elaborate testing, surgical, and research facilities. You may be paying for testing and treatment capabilities that you don't need for your basic diagnostic workup. Find out what they charge and compare their rates to what other doctors charge in your community.

Many communities are not large enough to support fertility specialists and in vitro clinics. Traveling to distant medical facilities may add unnecessarily to your out-of-pocket expenses, absenteeism from work, and overall level of stress. If you have a good family practitioner and/or OB-GYN in your community who knows quite a bit about fertility treatment, I'd encourage you to begin there rather than travel hundreds of miles to a stranger. The "expert" isn't necessarily better just because he or she is located over one hundred miles away.

A Final Note About Selecting a Doctor

Fertility treatment isn't magic. It is a structured, organized investigation. An obstetrician-gynecologist working together with a urologist can diagnose and successfully treat the majority of people with fertility problems. Ultimately you should judge any doctor's ability based on the treatment plan he or she outlines especially for you and on the doctor's responsiveness to your problems and concerns.

Making a List and Checking It Twice

The first interview with your doctor provides an excellent opportunity for you to assess how well you will be able to work together.

To prepare for your first visit, write down a list of questions you want to ask. To help formulate your questions, you may want to refer to the following list of questions people most frequently ask me.

If you are already receiving fertility treatment, it is not too late to ask your doctor these questions. If you spot any of the "Four Poor Treatment Danger Signs" discussed below, you may wish to reconsider your choice of doctor(s).

Questions to Ask Your Doctor

About the Doctor's Practice

Do you have experience in fertility treatment?

Will you refer me to an obstetrician when I get pregnant or will you deliver the baby?

Will you send me to any other physician or laboratories for treatments or tests?

Will you treat my spouse? If not, who will?

Do you arrange for adoptions?

Do you document surgeries with photographs or videotapes so I can see your findings for myself or provide them to other doctors?

Which hospital(s) do you use?

Do you use Pergonal to induce ovulation? If so, do you monitor egg development with ultrasound to avoid multiple births?

Do you perform sterilization reversals? What is your success rate? (Should be about 50 percent.)

Do you perform microsurgery? What is your success rate for vasectomy reversal? (Should be about 90 percent.) For fallopian tube repair? (Should be 50 to 70 percent.)

Do you belong to the American Fertility Society?

Are you on the RESOLVE, Inc., recommended list of physicians?

About Tests, Surgery, and Treatments

What kind of procedure is it?

What will the procedure tell you?

What results do you expect?

How long will it take?

What will it cost? Does insurance cover it?

Will it hurt?

How will it make me feel afterward?

Can you do it in your office? As a hospital outpatient?

Will I be incapacitated? For how long?

Will I miss work?

Will my spouse be involved? How? Will he/she miss work?

Can I drive home afterward?

How many times will it be repeated?

Will it interfere with our sex life? How?
Will we have to delay our vacation?

About Medications

What results do you expect?
How long/often will I take it?
What will it cost? Does insurance cover it?
Will it hurt or have side effects?
Do I take it at home or at your office?
Will I have to miss time at work?
How many times will it be repeated?
Will we have to delay our vacation?

Four Poor Treatment Danger Signs

Once you've selected your physician, *you are responsible for monitoring your doctor's performance*. That may sound strange to you, but if you hired a carpenter, auto mechanic, or roofer, you wouldn't think twice about making sure you were getting the work you contracted for. It's the same for a doctor. However, you must be an informed consumer in order to evaluate the doctor's performance.

Below are four danger signs that will alert you that you may have chosen the wrong person:

1. *No clear-cut fertility treatment plan.* If your physician does not formulate and discuss a treatment plan, you may be on the "hit-or-miss" regimen. After your first conference, your doctor should be able to outline the initial phases of your workup. After the basic workup, which may take four to six weeks, your doctor should be able to outline a treatment plan. You should be confident that your doctor, as would any good investigator, is using specific step-by-step procedures for getting answers about your fertility problem. If your doctor hasn't shared the plan with you, ask for a detailed explanation.

Take notes and make sure that your doctor follows that course. If your doctor deviates from the plan, find out why. Was it because of an unexpected test result? Did the doctor forget certain details that were planned initially? Remember, *ask questions when they arise*. Waiting for the straw that breaks the camel's back or assuming that the doctor is an infallible being who will take care of everything will get you into trouble. If your doctor's response to your request for a plan is not adequate, find a different doctor.

2. *Poor communication.* If you can't talk to your doctor, at least one of you has a problem. Doctors are usually very busy, so as a rule they won't sit down and strike up a conversation hoping that eventually you will feel at ease enough to ask a question. If, after you leave the doctor's office, you always remember a question you meant to ask, I encourage you to write down your questions before your appointments. You should feel free to call back and talk to the nurse practitioner or to the doctor personally. If you feel that your doctor is not taking your questions seriously, is giving you superficial answers, seems impatient about explaining terms and treatment, persistently talks over your head, will not return your calls, or is too frequently not available when you need help, find another.

3. *Unorthodox treatment or methods.* If your doctor deviates from orthodox regimes—for example, by failing to perform a semen analysis, prescribing fertility drugs before doing a complete fertility evaluation, or administering Pergonal without using an ultrasound to monitor the number of eggs you're developing—you have reason to be concerned.

Talk to your physician. Don't just assume he or she is incompetent. You may have misunderstood something you heard or read, or your condition might be out of the ordinary. If after getting the doctor's answers you are still troubled, however, you may wish to request a second opinion, especially when surgery is recommended. No good doctor should balk at this perfectly reasonable request. If you don't think your doctor is using the "best" fertility treatment procedures or if you lack faith in your doctor's decisions, then find another doctor.

4. *Your Treatment is taking too long.* This is a tough one because the amount of time required to diagnose and treat each fertility problem is different for each patient. However, there are a few benchmarks you can watch for. Your initial workup should be complete within four to six weeks—two months at most. At that point your doctor should be able to give you the preliminary findings and should present your options for additional tests or treatment.

As your treatment progresses, you may tend to become impatient. You may forget, for example, that even after you are "cured," you are no more fertile than the average population at your age. At the most, you have a 20 percent chance of getting pregnant each month. So if your doctor feels that your fertility problem is resolved after six months of treatment, it may take another six to nine months for you to get pregnant. If you don't conceive in that time, your doctor may recommend conducting further tests.

Doctors may often use a more aggressive treatment approach with an older couple like Richard and Margaret B., who were in their mid-thirties. A woman in that age group doesn't have that many fertile years left, and her odds for "normal" pregnancy are getting slimmer each year. If you feel your fertile years are slipping away, discuss your concerns with your doctor. If your doctor isn't responsive, find another doctor.

I tailor the rate of treatment to each couple. Some people want to know all of the answers *right now*. Others want to proceed more slowly—they need time for things to sink in. For example, Shelley T. had a limited budget, so the pacing of her treatment plan was slower than for Margaret, who wanted to get pregnant as soon as possible. Each of these women required a custom-designed treatment plan that would accommodate her life style.

Is your treatment taking too long? That's very hard to judge. But if you're really worried about it, talk with your doctor and your RESOLVE support group counselors. *If you don't feel that you're making progress, get a second opinion or find a new doctor.*

I encourage you to learn as much as you can about fertility treatment and, above all, never to accept your doctor's recommendations complacently. Ultimately, *you* are responsible for the quality of care you receive. You are responsible for selecting the doctor who is best qualified to help you get your miracle baby.

By *Mark Perloe and Linda Gail Christie*

New Infertility Treatment Is Done In Doctor's Office

A new procedure performed in a doctor's office should eventually allow thousands of infertile American women to become pregnant without major surgery, a team of radiologists reported in San Francisco.

The report not only seems to herald a low-cost and safe method of helping women with blocked fallopian tubes, but it also highlights a growing turf battle spurred by money and professional rivalry that has erupted lately between radiologists and other medical specialists.

Historically, radiologists' main task has been to take pictures with X-rays so surgeons and others could plan therapy. Already among the highest paid of doctors, radiologists now are flexing new high-technology muscles and taking business from other physicians. The tools that let them see inside the body increasingly let them fix what they find wrong.

The example of the growing power of radiology came from Dr. Amy Suzanne Thurmond of the Oregon Health Sciences University in Portland, Oregon, who described her new technique for treating fertility at the meeting of the American Roentgen Ray Society.

Some 2,000 radiologists who use X-rays, ultrasound, magnetic fields, and other technologies to image the inside of the body attended sessions on a wide range of medical topics.

Tools Threaded Through Catheter

Developed in the last three years, the method she described relies on a catheter, a long flexible tube through which specialized tools can be threaded. It is similar to catheters used by radiologists and other physicians to put dye in arteries to see whether they are blocked, and often to clear the blockages. The doctor guides the tube through the vagina and uterus and into the fallopian tubes, using an X-ray machine to watch its progress.

Thurmond said blocked fallopian tubes, which carry eggs from the ovaries to the uterus, account for 10 to 25 percent of infertility in American women.

Blockages are cleared in either of two ways, Thurmond said. The first step is to inject, under pressure, a dye monitored with X-ray imaging equipment. The fluid by itself may clear the tube, which the doctor can see on the X-ray screen. If that doesn't work, a small, flexible wire narrower than a paper clip is projected from the end of the catheter, puncturing its way through the obstacle.

The technique also allows doctors to determine whether eggs are blocked by spasms in the walls of the fallopian tubes, or by physical obstacles.

The method has been tried on fifty women. In thirty-two, the tubes were opened successfully. As of last week, eleven of the women had gotten pregnant. The success rate, Thurmond said, is equal to or better than traditional surgery.

Importantly, the new method costs only about 400 dollars, requires no hospitalization, and takes less than an hour. It is experimental now, but can be done in a doctor's office.

In contrast, standard surgery to correct blocked fallopian tubes by opening up the abdomen for access is not only more risky, but also typically costs 9,000 dollars and requires several days' hospitalization and several weeks for full recovery.

Bumping Fields

The new method is a perfect illustration of how new equipment wielded by radiologists bumps them against fields traditionally dominated by other medical specialists. A new specialty with its own organization and journals has even arisen, called "interventional radiology."

Radiologists circulate pamphlets that describe how they can use catheters and similar devices to block bloodflow to tumors, clear arteries, and drain abscesses in internal organs, all without the help of a surgeon.

"We were supposed to be a service for other doctors," said Dr. Lee F. Rogers, incoming president of the society and chairman of the radiology department at Northwestern University Medical School in Illinois. "Now we're getting more aggressive. It's a turf battle."

Partly in response, members of other specialties are adopting the catheters and other radiological tools in hopes of holding on to a changing business.

For example, the fallopian tube-clearing method closely resembles a method announced earlier by a gynecological surgeon, Dr. Norbert Gleicher of Mount Sinai Hospital Medical Center in Chicago. He, too, uses a catheter to clear blocked tubes but adds an inflatable balloon at the tip to expand tubes in hopes that they will stay clear longer.

Reached by telephone, Gleicher said his method and Thurmond's are "fully compatible," and he praised her work. He expects both sets of tools to be employed in a combined fashion when the method reached general use, probably in a few years after extensive trials are completed to prove safety and effectiveness.

By *Charles Petit*

Donor Insemination—Traditions and Techniques

Indications for Donor Insemination

It has been pointed out that the ease of DI has directed attention and research away from understanding and treating male infertility. This is in contrast to the aggressive and prolific treatment of female infertility, which is much more interventionist because of the internal placement of the female reproductive organs.

Yet it is precisely the untreatable nature of male infertility, as Achilles observed, that makes it an indication for DI. Although euphemistically termed a "treatment," it does not alter the infertility of the male, and the female is, of course, presumed to be fertile.

One cynic commented that "there are no indications for DI, only requests." We will now look at the reasons why DI is performed.

1. *Primary infertility*. Many of the causes of male infertility, if not medically resolved, become indications for DI.

2. *Eugenics*. In these cases sperm production may be normal, but there is a hereditary or familial disease, which the male does not want to reproduce. Twenty percent of DI nationwide is done for genetic factors; for example, genetic diseases such as Huntington's disease, Klinefelter's syndrome, Hoffmann's disease, and muscular dystrophy. Some diseases, like von Recklinghausen's disease and Huntington's chorea, have variable expressions and do not show up until midlife. Donor insemination, of course, does not eliminate genetic risk, it simply reduces it. For example, with Werdnig-Hoffmann disease or cystic disease of the pancreas, the risk is still one percent, but that is much better than 25 percent. Also, prenatal screening can be done, such as amniocentesis, and alphafetoprotein blood tests.

3. *Immunological reasons*. The most common situation is when there is incompatibility between a woman and her male partner's Rh factor. Sometimes a woman's cervical mucus becomes "hostile" and causes an immune response to her partner's sperm. (Donor cervical mucus can be tried, too, and mucus can be successfully stored for a few weeks at four degrees centigrade.)

4. *Vasectomy and remarriage*. This is an increasingly common indication for DI and accounted for 12 percent of inseminations nationwide when surveyed by Curie-Cohen, et al., in 1980. In California, vasectomy is now more often the reason for DI than primary infertility.

History of Donor Insemination

Donor insemination was the first step of a whole range of reproductive assistance that is available today. Its history goes back centuries. As early as 220 A.D., the Talmud questioned the paternity of a child who was born after a woman was accidentally fertilized in bath water. In the thirteenth century, there is documentation of a rabbi's concern about the fertilization of a woman sleeping on bed linen where a man had ejaculated.

The history of donor insemination in animals is more documented than human donor insemination. Arabs in the fourteenth century used techniques of artificial insemination in breeding horses. A wad of wool was first placed in a mare's vagina and then under the nose of a stallion, who ejaculated in response. The wad of wool, which caught the semen, was then placed in the mare, who became with foal. The story goes that a sheik even inseminated his enemy's pure mares with semen from diseased inferior stallions. Varasotto, in the same century, artificially inseminated sheep. Don Ponchom, a monk in the abbey of Reame, wrote about experimental fertilization with fish eggs. The existence of spermatozoa was discovered under the microscope by the Dutchman Anton van Leeuwenhoek in 1677, but he did not know their function.

Bartholomeus Eustachius, in 1550, advised using a finger to guide semen toward the opening of the uterus after intercourse and, in 1779, the Italian priest and physiologist Lazaro Spallanzani artificially inseminated reptiles and dogs and observed the effects of freezing on human sperm. Around 1790 John Hunter of London first recorded a pregnancy and delivery of a child conceived by artificial insemination with a husband's semen. In 1838, the Frenchman Girault blew sperm into the vagina via a hollow tube. In 1865, a pamphlet on artificial insemination was published by De Haut in France, but he discontinued his experimentation due to great public outcry. In the late nineteenth century Marion Sims, an American gynecologist, reported fifty-five artificial inseminations that he performed on six women. The success rate of his "ethereal copulation" (he used ether on the women) was only 4 percent because he thought that menstruation indicated ovulation. The first reported successful artificial insemination (with husband's semen) in the United States occurred in 1866. That same year the concept of sperm banks was originated by Mantagazzi. De Lajotre, in 1876, claimed a success rate of 88 percent with 567 women by using their husband's semen. He was later condemned by the Tribunal of Bordeaux for doubtful practices.

In 1884, Dr. William Pancoast, of Jefferson Medical College in Philadelphia, first documented a successful donor insemination. (The accuracy of this well-known story has been questioned.) Dr. Pancoast anesthetized the wife of an infertile man and used semen from the most handsome man in his class of medical students. He did not inform either the husband or wife of his action, which, as Gena Corea points out in *The Mother Machine*, makes his act a rape. After the birth of the child, the doctor did confess his secret to the husband, who reportedly received the news with great enthusiasm.

One must also wonder about the nature of the prior physical examination which Hard (1909), one of Pancoast's medical students, described as "very complete, almost as perfect as any army examination." The author continues, "As a matter of possible public interest, I will say that during this examination was discovered for the first time, as far as I know, the suction function of the uterus which takes place during orgasm." Hard subsequently visited the world's first recorded artificially conceived offspring, by then a businessman in New York.

Clearly, the potential of DI loomed large in Hard's vision at the beginning of the century, as he expressed in the following amazing diatribe:

> From a nature point of view, the idea of artificial impregnation offers valuable advantages. The mating of human beings must, from the nature of things, be a matter of sentiment alone. Persons

of the worst possible promise of good and healthy offspring are being lawfully united in marriage every day. Marriage is a proposition which is not submitted to good judgment or even common sense, as a rule. No Burbank methods are possible, even tho [sic] they be ideal. Artificial impregnation by carefully selected seed, alone will solve the problem. It may at first shock the delicate sensibilities of the sentimental who consider that the source of the seed indicates the true father, but when the scientific fact becomes known that the origin of the spermatozoa which generates the ovum is of no more importance than the personality of the finger which pulls the trigger of a gun, then objections will lose their forcefulness and artificial impregnation become recognized as a race-uplifting procedure.

It is gradually becoming well establist [sic] that the mother is the complete builder of the child. It is her blood that gives it material for its body and her nerve energy which is divided to supply its vital force. It is her mental ideals which go to influence, to some extent at least, the features, the tendencies, and the mental caliber of the child. "Many a man rocks another man's child and thinks he is rocking his own" for it looks like him. And often two children by the same parents have features entirely dissimilar. It is the predominating mental ideals prevailing with the mother that shapes the destiny of the child. The man who thrusts his nose into a beautiful blossom to surfeit his sense of smell on the sweet perfume, is merely breathing the lustful odor from the sexual organ of the plant; and if his nose displaces some of the pollen, he may be the father of the next flower. If a honey bee does the work, it might be called the father.

A scientific study of sex selection without regard to marriage conditions, might result in giving some men children of wonderful mental endowments, in place of half-witted, evil-inclined, disease-disposed offspring which they are ashamed to call their own. The mechanical method of impregnation, whether it be the orthodox way of the aseptic surgeon's skillful fingers, counts but little,

> except sentiment, and sentiment is fast becoming a servant instead of a master in the affairs of the human race. Few are the children that are brought intentionally into this world. As a rule they are but the incidental result of a journey in search of selfish pleasure. They are seldom sought, and often unwelcome when they put in their first appearance. The subsequent mother's love is largely a matter of growth, for affection is but an attribute of selfishness.
>
> The man who may think this idea shocking probably has millions of gonococci swarming in his seminal ducts, and probably his wife has had a laparotomy which nearly cost her life itself, as a result of his infecting her with the crop reaped from his last planting of "wild oats."

Hard closes with an indictment of the prevalence of venereal disease at the time.

In 1907, Ivanoff, a physiologist, wrote that there were real advantages in using artificial insemination on a large scale in animal husbandry. In fact, techniques, protocols, and legal lineage (the donor is always the sire) of DI in animals have been much more highly developed than for humans.

By the early 1900s, the practice of DI was well under way. Twenty-four articles had been written on the subject of DI in the United States by 1938, and a 1941 survey estimated that almost 3,700 inseminations had occurred in the United States. In the 1980s, estimates range from 10,000 to 100,000 DI children per year; the state of California alone may have 20,000 annually. The numbers are vague because of the secrecy around the procedure. It is estimated that there are over one million DI offspring in the United States, with thousands around the world as well. Yugoslavia, for example, has an estimated 5,000 a year, England and Australia over 2,000, Switzerland and Denmark over 1,000, and over 300 and rising in Sweden despite that country's recent legislation, which protects the child's right to know her paternal origin.

Definitions

Artificial insemination is a technique whereby semen is placed in the vagina, cervical canal, or uterus by means other than sexual intercourse, for the purpose of inducing pregnancy. Because of the association with animal husbandry and to avoid acknowledging the donor, other terms have been suggested such as alternative, therapeutic, or even abnormal fertilization.

Husband Insemination

AIH is artificial insemination with the husband's semen, in contrast to AID—artificial insemination by donor, or DI as we now call it. It is also known as "endogenous" or "homologous" insemination. This is done when some mechanical difficulty prevents the husband from depositing the semen in his wife's vagina—such as impotence, hypospadias (semen lost through a congenital opening on the underside of the penis), or retrograde ejaculation (semen enters the bladder). There may be physical deformities, paralysis, or psychological conditions that also prevent natural insemination.

When oligospermia (less than thirty million sperm) is present, several semen samples may be taken and pooled to increase the concentration of sperm. A centrifuge technique spins the sperm for a couple of minutes. The first portion of an ejaculator ("split ejaculate") is used as it contains less prostatic fluid and thus a higher concentration of sperm. The concentration of sperm seems to be more important than the total number of sperm. Laboratory screening to eliminate abnormal sperm and other debris in the semen by passing it through a nylon membrane may also increase the possibility of conception.

Cervical mucus that is "hostile" to a partner's sperm may be receptive to the sperm from a donor. In such cases, there is a definite body-mind link to be explored. Psychological aids, such as visualization, can help, but it is probably necessary to understand the "hostility" of the mucus first. It is interesting that when the mucus and semen are mixed together prior to AIH, the success rate is doubled (from 21 to 42 percent).

Shapiro (1981) cites a case where a woman was allergic to her husband's semen, developing shortness of breath and hives if a condom were not used or if it leaked. She also had positive skin tests to semen from vasectomized men (who have no sperm in their semen). After seven cycles of AIH, with sperm only, she successfully conceived and delivered twins. There is another case of a woman who developed an allergic reaction to her husband's semen during pregnancy. The authors observe the "immunologic potential of human coitus," which is clearly psychosomatic.

Donor Insemination

DI is artificial insemination with semen from a donor and is also known as "exogamous" or "heterologous," "therapeutic," or "aided" insemination. Some prefer the more technical names because AID stresses the major drawbacks of the procedure—the artificiality and the presence of a donor.

Semen obtained from one donor may be used for many impregnations and can be kept indefinitely through freezing and storage in sperm banks. When two or more inseminations are done in one cycle, different donors may be used for each attempt. However, Langer et al. (1969) in Israel refused subsequent DI unless the same donor was used.

Although the procedure may be helpful, safe, and painless, concern is rarely expressed for the consequences of the procedure.

In a couple relationship with male infertility, DI (in contrast with AIH) introduces a third party. Traditionally the donor's identity is highly guarded, in order to protect the donor and physician. Single or lesbian women may also place secrecy at a premium for their own protection against a possible paternity suit.

Mixed Insemination

AIM refers to the practice of mixing the husband's and donor's semen. It is also know as AIHD or CAI, confused artificial insemination; BAI, biseminal artificial insemination; the "French firing squad" technique; or, in German, the "pathfinders' action." Although the Curie-Cohen survey found that 15 percent of physicians mixed semen, only ignorant physicians would recommend it today. Even Guttmacher (1962) protested:

> I feel that if the couple cannot face the reality of the fact that this will be a child of the seed of an unrelated man, then I think they are not intellectually and emotionally ripe for the procedure. Therefore I have not been tempted to lull them into a kind of feeling that this might still be the husband's child.

Before the days of blood tests, Finegold suggested that AIM could provide the means for a court to presume in favor of the husband's paternity.

The rationale that practitioners give for AIM is that the husband may then let himself believe that by a remote chance he might be the biological father. It could be argued that this procedure would make it even harder for the husband to accept DI under these circumstances, where his own chances of biological fatherings were not ruled out. Also, the use of AIM implies that the husband's infertility is marginal, if such a conception is at all possible. Therefore, one might ask, why is donor semen being used?

Some physicians mix the sperm from different donors, again to confuse the issue of paternity. Any mixing of sperm offers no advantage for improving the chances of conception and, in fact, may have an adverse effect on the semen. More important, AIM for the purpose of confusing the records to preserve donor anonymity is ethically unacceptable but often practiced by lesbians and single women to avoid future paternity suits.

Techniques of Insemination

As Stephen Steigrad, a Sydney gynecologist, puts it, "The actual technique of artificial insemination is one of life's great non-events." This is why self-insemination is so simple.

Masturbation is the usual way of obtaining a semen specimen for artificial insemination, and sperm obtained this way remain mobile longer. However, semen can be collected in a number of other ways: 1) *Coitus.* Retrieval of semen from a condom or even from the vagina after coitus interruptus; 2) *Surgical biopsy* of the testicle or epididymis; or, 3) *Postmortem* because sperm production is the last body function to cease.

The semen must be used within two hours, and it can be introduced by several different techniques.

1. *Intravaginal.* The semen is simply deposited in the vagina with a syringe, straw in an applicator, test tube, the lower blade of a plastic speculum, or even a turkey baster. Metal is not used because it has a spermicidal effect.

2. *Applied to the cervix* in a rubber contraceptive cervical cap, plastic insemination cup, diaphragm, or sponge.

3. *Intracervical application* with a cannula if the opening to the cervix is narrowed (stenosis of the external os). It is important that only a small amount of semen be used, a quarter of a milliliter or less, and that it be introduced very slowly into the cervix so that it does not enter the uterus.

Otherwise, cramps can occur from the prostaglandins in the semen. Also, many more abnormal sperm (if not screened) reach the uterus than normally would if they had to make their way through the acidic vaginal secretions. This can lead to infections such as an abscess, endometritis (inflammation of the lining of the uterus), or even peritonitis (inflammation within the abdominal cavity). However, some practitioners, such as Neil Barwin in Ottawa, Canada, routinely do intracervical inseminations, and report only rare side effects, three cases in four hundred requiring transient hospitalization.

Selection of Women

In the overwhelming majority of inseminations in the United States, the gynecologist simply uses his own judgment in treating couples or single women with DI. In other countries, a team approach—combining physician, social worker, or psychologist—is more usual. The role is not always selection, but rather presenting information and alternatives so that individuals can drop out themselves, if they so choose. Sometimes such teams are recommended, not to supply objective advice about the unknown outcome of DI, but merely as a means of reducing any possible criticism of the selection process. In fact, I personally know social workers who have left such teams because of conflicts with other members over the issues of secrecy and disclosure to the child.

Each clinic and physician will have their policies of exclusion—no single women, no women over forty, or whatever—which have made sperm banks that market directly to the consumer a popular alternative. The larger the institution, generally, the longer the waiting list and the more structured the routine.

Determining Ovulation

The most important aspect of donor insemination is timing. The egg is viable for less than twenty-four hours, although sperm survival is longer—up to days. It is crucial, then, to determine the time of ovulation. Usually women are required to take their basal body temperature (BBT) on waking for three months to observe their ovulation pattern.

If conception has not occurred within six months of DI, then clinical investigations of ovulation may be begun, which might include systemic tests, such as thyroid function. There are also other unrecognized and poorly defined conditions that affect the success of insemination.

Ovulation can be estimated by radioimmune assay blood tests (which are slow) or rapid LH estimates (which are not always sufficiently sensitive) to check for that hormone peak. Ultrasound scans of the ovaries reveal the status of the ripening egg follicle and reliably can predict or observe ovulation. However, ultrasound scans are expensive, and one to five of them may be necessary until the main follicle ruptures. Other assessments of ovulation include examining the cervical mucus under the microscope (between days eleven and thirteen) for certain qualities found at the time of ovulation such as a "ferning" pattern of crystallization, stretchiness ("Spinnbarkheit"), and the absence of cells. Sometimes estrogen is prescribed for seven to ten days of the cycle to improve the quality and quantity of the cervical mucus because it is very important for conception. Levels of plasma progesterone can be estimated between days twenty-one and twenty-four and confirm whether ovulation has occurred.

However, many practitioners find that it is "more effective" to induce ovulation rather than to predict it. It is not uncommon for the many women undergoing DI to have treatment with clomiphene citrate (known as Clomid or Serophene), which induces ovulation. It is thus used to produce a predictable ovulation, even though a 1981 study found that the use of clomiphene meant less than a one-day shift of the predicted day of ovulation. This medication is prescribed for failure to ovulate as well as poor function in the luteal, or postovulation phase, of the cycle. It can also stabilize irregular cycles. The decreased function in previously ovulating women is a reaction to the stress of DI. So many women (30 to 67 percent of reported studies) fail to ovulate at some time while undergoing DI that the term "DI-induced anovulation" has arisen. The menstrual clock of the hypothalamus in the brain can be affected by stress due to time off work, travel, expense, or ambivalence about being impregnated with a stranger's sperm. This drug is actually an antiestrogen and it may decrease the amount of ovulation mucus, so that estrogen is often prescribed as well. Clomid is given in doses of 50 to 150 milligrams a day for five days beginning on the fifth day of the cycle. This will cause ovulation about six days after the last pill, i.e., on day sixteen. There are also side effects from Clomid, such as swelling and possible cysts of the ovaries. Also, the chance of multiple pregnancy is increased when more than one egg is stimulated for release at ovulation. Some doctors, tired of a guessing game each month, will give 5,000 to 10,000 units of HCG (human chorionic gonadotropin, a potent "fertility drug") at midcycle, which will produce ovulation within forty-eight hours. However, Federation CECOS in France (1983) cites a study that implicates inducers of ovulation as a cause of chromosomal abnormalities.

Female Infertility Workup

Many clinics will do six months of DI on the basis of a woman's BBT charts, which show evidence of ovulation. However, some physicians insist on a comprehensive workup, or fertility examination, from the outset. While this may be cost-effective for the physician, it usually isn't for the patient. However, if a woman has not conceived after a few months, it may make sense to undergo some investigations, including psychological counseling. Of course, the woman must also be in good general health and not suffer from such conditions as diabetes or heart disease.

One of the simplest tests is the post-coital test (PCT) to check for survival and motility of the sperm in the cervical mucus. Around days twelve to fourteen, not later than ovulation, and within two to six hours after insemination, some mucus is aspirated from the cervix and examined under the microscope. Prior to insemination, a drop of semen can be placed on a microscope with some cervical mucus to check for compatibility, too. Any infection (cervicitis) will be indicated by the presence of white blood cells and can be observed at this time and treated.

A hysterosalpingogram (HSG) is an X-ray to check if the fallopian tubes are open. A dye is injected into the uterus so that any blockages in the tubes can be observed (and occasionally cleared by the procedure). The HSG has virtually replaced the Rubin or insufflation test, which checked patency of the tubes with carbon dioxide. If the patient felt shoulder pain then this was an indication that the gas had passed into the abdominal cavity and that the tubes were open. Broekhuizen (1980) observed that where routine HSGs were done on women undergoing DI, 80 percent were unnecessary.

A diagnostic laparoscopy is an investigation of the reproductive organs through the abdomen, under anesthesia. It requires an incision so small that this operation has been dubbed "Band-Aid surgery." The abdomen is distended with gas, usually carbon dioxide, to make the organs easier to see through a lighted telescope. Using the laparoscope, the physician can determine whether the tubes are open or closed, whether scar tissue is interfering with the movement and function of the tubes, and whether tubal surgery is necessary. The ovary can be viewed directly to determine whether it is functioning normally. If necessary, a biopsy of the ovary can be taken for examination, or eggs can be collected for examination, testing, or for in vitro fertilization. The HSG and diagnostic laparoscopy are performed during days five to thirteen of the menstrual cycle, after bleeding has stopped and before ovulation.

An endometrial biopsy involves scraping a small piece of the lining of the uterus, prior to menstruation, to examine it for hormone changes that would indicate ovulation. This procedure also proves that the cervical canal is sufficiently open.

Number of Inseminations Per Cycle

The Curie-Cohen survey (1979) found that 17 percent of practitioners did one insemination per cycle, 61.4 percent did two, and 20.5 percent did three inseminations per cycle. More inseminations are done with frozen than fresh semen because sperm vigor is reduced by freezing. Interestingly, the success rates were independent of the number of times women were inseminated in a single cycle or the timing with which inseminations were spaced. The only significant factor was the size of the doctor's practice, the larger practices having higher success rates.

Multiple inseminations are typically done on the day before, the day of, and the day after ovulation. Day zero is the last day of the lowest point of the temperature (nadir) before the rise. Some say this is the best day, other practitioners found it better either the day before or the day after. DI is sometimes done every other day. Another opinion is that a single insemination per cycle means better timing, with less expense (75 to 100 dollars per insemination) and wastage of sperm, and has equivalent or better results. A 1980 study by Propping, in West Germany, showed multiple inseminations to be only half as effective as single ones. The explanation put forth is that a second insemination may disturb a pregnancy that has already resulted.

Fifty-one percent of Curie-Cohen's respondents used the same donor for each insemination of a single cycle, but different donors for each cycle, whereas 31.8 percent used different donors within a single cycle.

Results of Donor Insemination

The success of DI is calculated in many different ways. Fecundability means the probability of conception in a menstrual cycle, and fertility refers to the actual conception. Higher rates of success are usually reported with fresh rather than frozen semen. However, patient selection, insemination techniques, number of cycles, and the follow-up of the results of DI are not uniform. Some writers calculate the successful pregnancies according to the incidence of pregnancies per cycle and others total the overall pregnancy rate (the ratio of conceptions to patients receiving DI). This latter rate varies with the number of women who do not complete the advised regimen (losses to follow-up) either because they dropped out or were still hoping to conceive on the program when the data were analyzed. The rate of conception usually refers to the frequency or percentage of conceptions achieved in a certain cycle. The cumulative rate shows the distribution of conceptions by the number of cycles required for conception. This proportion uses as its denominator only those women who conceived and ignores women who did not conceive. Such a proportion does not represent the probability that a woman will conceive by a certain cycle, because it is conditional on a pregnancy being actually achieved.

The cumulative rate of conception obtained by life-table analysis takes into consideration the experience of all the women on the DI program. The life-table method corrects for variable periods of follow-up and losses to follow-up, as it has been argued that dropouts should be classified as failures. The life-table analysis estimates what conception rates would have been had all patients completed a specific number of DI cycles, and thus provides a true measure of the chance of conception.

Nowhere has the success of DI been 100 percent, and the national average, according to Curie-Cohen's survey (1979), was 57 percent. Worldwide rates range from 40 to 80 percent. Guttmacher reported an average of 69 percent in 1962. The highest success rates are in the first three or four cycles, by which time about one-third have conceived. Some practitioners claim that pregnancy rates fall off after the first few months and then about two-thirds of women drop out of the program. Successful clinics have cumulative pregnancy rates of up to 85 percent of those women who persist for a year or longer, using life-table analysis. Glezerman reported that 98 percent of women conceived within thirteen cycles. A study by Bergquist et al. at Johns Hopkins Hospital in Baltimore, published in 1982, concluded that "patients can be advised that their chance of conception with DI should approach that of normal fertile couples." They studied 226 women, using fresh semen, usually two inseminations per cycle, with the cervical cup technique. Using a mathematical model of cumulative pregnancy rates, their rate was 62.5 percent after six months and for those who continued to undergo DI beyond six months the monthly probability of pregnancy did not decline. By ten months, 82.4 percent of patients had conceived. (With natural insemination, about 30 percent conceive within the first three months, 50 percent by six months, and 80 percent by the end of a year.)

Glezerman and White (1981) describe the ideal DI patient as a woman who is younger than thirty-five, belongs to a higher socioeconomic class, has suffered less than seven years of infertility, has no ovulatory disturbance, and has sufficient emotional support from her male partner. In fact, his study found that only 28.6 percent of women whose partners did not accompany them for the inseminations achieved pregnancy, compared with 98.6 percent of those whose partners did. There was a higher abortion rate also in the unaccompanied women, and more than 70 percent of them discontinued DI with or without notification. The absence of the male partner at inseminations was interpreted as resistance, despite his formal acceptance of DI as evidenced by the signed agreement.

An interesting comment on the female factor in fertility was reported by Emperaire, et al. (1980), in the British medical journal *Lancet*. If the male partner's sperm count was zero, 96 percent of the women undergoing DI became pregnant within six months. However, if he had a count of zero to twenty million, only 70 percent of the women did. Likewise, Albrecht (1982) in Boston found a 20 percent fecundability in women with azoospermic partners compared with 10 percent for those whose men were merely oligospermic. They interpreted this to mean that women married to men with low sperm counts are a selected population with subnormal fertility and are unable to compensate for the deficient sperm counts of their husbands. One could also postulate that DI is more acceptable when there is absolutely no hope of conception with one's husband, and that this has a psychological effect on the woman's fertility.

Levie (1967) found that four previously infertile husbands showed a "spontaneous remission" of their infertility after their wives had already delivered DI offspring. Each of these men were apparently able to "beget" a child.

Age

Most practitioners find that fertility drops when the woman reaches thirty or thirty-five. Decreased fertility over age thirty-five is often due to the pathology of the pelvic organs. Peak fecundability has been estimated at age twenty-four. Others, like Chong and Taymor, reported (1975) that there was no age effect on fertility. Cesarean rates, which are higher in births resulting from reproductive technologies ("the premium baby") are further elevated in older women.

Fresh or Frozen Semen

Frozen semen was used by 31.4 percent of the Curie-Cohen respondents but accounted for only 12.7 percent of total donor semen. Of those who used frozen semen, 43.7 percent used it in less than 10 percent of their inseminations, and 41.2 percent used it in an average of 90 percent of them. The use of frozen semen was independent of the size of the practice and the size of the population served. Even more striking was the fact that the use of frozen semen was independent of whether the physician treated a woman with the same donor for every cycle or different donors within a single cycle.

Of those physicians who used frozen semen, 87 percent never stored it over two years, and 68 percent obtained outside donors. Of those who never or rarely used frozen semen, only 8 percent used donors from outside their own geographic area.

Usually, twice as many inseminations are required for frozen as fresh semen, but some practitioners feel the advantages outweigh its lower pregnancy rate. A study done by Kovacs and Lording in Melbourne, Australia in 1980 involved 252 patients who used frozen semen and, with at least two inseminations per cycle, had less successful results. The life-table pregnancy rates were 47.6 percent after six months and 62.8 percent after twelve months. However, another Melbourne study by Clayton in 1980 showed that 50 percent conceived within three cycles and 85 percent by six months.

As a result of AIDS, frozen semen only is recommended by the American Association of Tissue Banks, the Center for Disease Control, and the Food and Drug Administration. In Australia, guidelines require the use of fresh semen. Freezing semen allows it to be quarantined (currently for ninety days), but some banks follow the Australian standard of six months), pending a blood test of the donor to clear him of AIDS antibodies. With such guidelines, a physician who uses fresh semen may be at increased risk for malpractice by not adhering to "standards of practice." Thus, sperm banks report increased demand; as one said, "Cleared semen is like liquid gold," and customers are reserving it several months in advance.

When a test for the AIDS *antigen* is developed, quarantining, which allows time for the *antibody* response to the antigen, will no longer be necessary. The American Fertility Society guidelines (October 1986) indicate that fresh semen is safe if their screening procedures are followed (although some AFS members disagree). The majority of physicians are continuing to use fresh semen, according to most sources.

Spontaneous Abortion (Miscarriage) Rate

The rate of miscarriage following DI is no different from natural conception. Numbers range from 8.9 percent in an Australian study to 10.7 percent in a report from Baltimore. Chong and Taymor found the miscarriage rate higher among women aged thirty to thirty-nine compared with those aged twenty to twenty-nine.

Congenital Malformations

Reports of congenital anomalies among DI offspring are less than those naturally conceived, which is 2 to 3 percent. This may be a result of underreporting, although one study looked out for this and concluded that DI parents are more likely to report evident malformations. While the overall incidence of malformations may be lower in DI offspring, the incidence of chromosomal abnormalities may be increased (Fraser and Forse, 1981; Chong and Taymor, 1975; King and Magenis, 1978). Possibly these abnormalities result from stimulating ovulation.

The Sex Ratio of DI Offspring

Although there are reports in the literature that state no statistical difference in the genders of DI offspring, certainly the majority of studies show a much higher number of males than occurs naturally. Kleegman (1954) found that 70 percent were males when the DI occurred within twenty-four hours of ovulation, and 70 percent were females if the DI was done more than thirty-six hours after ovulation. Edvinsson (1983) in Sweden reported fifty males to thirty-six females.

Hazards for the DI Consumer

Often, infertile couples or single women, unless they contact a sperm bank directly, are obliged to place their trust in the physician they consult. Indeed, Lauerson and Ukane, in the November 1982 issue of *Cosmopolitan*, go so far as to say that "your knowledge and trust in your doctor are often essential for a successful conception." Belief surely does play a vital role in health and illness. However, couples are mostly unaware that their physician, if using frozen semen, has no control over the selection and screening of donors or the process of sperm preservation. For example, one of the substances used in cryobanking of semen is Tris, which is used to fireproof fabrics and has been found to be carcinogenic.

The problem with semen brokers, be they your gynecologist or an out-of-state sperm bank, is that the recipient is never 100 percent sure of the semen. Slome, writing in 1973 in the *British Medical Journal*, said that his personal experience with DI makes it difficult to suggest a sperm bank because the sperm can't be confirmed. The more parties involved, the more chance of confusion and error. Mail-order sperm can suffer a number of calamities en route. Although I have seen how they prepare, divide, and code the semen, like any bookkeeping system, there are bound to be mistakes. Straws will be misplaced, erroneously labeled, or broken. I have watched technicians in small crowded rooms, chatting away, with the radio blaring, dropping items on the floor, as they casually perform the freezing regimen.

Obviously, elaborate coding systems have been devised to minimize error, with different containers for different sperm. Some clinics have the patient fill in the records for matching the donor so that at least secretarial errors in transcription are avoided. Such doubts never arise when working with a donor friend, and the sperm comes fresh and pure.

The demand for DI can be expected to continually increase with media publicity, the rising incidence of male infertility, fewer infants available for adoption, more women (single, lesbian) wanting to bear a child without a male partner, and progress in genetic screening.

By *Elizabeth Noble*

SECTION 6

The Third Stairstep: The High-Tech Approach to Infertility

Introduction

The medical industry has never been reluctant or shy about touting its own inventions, particularly when those most involved are females. Thus, the procedure called in vitro fertilization/embryo transfer (IVF/ET) has been hailed as a panacea by physicians.

There are risks as well as benefits to IVF/ET, as is shown in pooled data from programs around the world. Well recognized is the risk of general anesthesia associated with laparoscopy, the surgical procedure used to retrieve eggs and/or diagnose female infertility problems like endometriosis.

New procedures—UDOR (ultrasonically directed oocyte [early stage of ovum before maturation] retrieval) and TUDOR (transabdominal/transvesical retrieval)—use local and regional anesthesia and are done on an outpatient basis; however, threading a needle through the vagina, bladder, or abdomen, to aspirate eggs, using ultrasound as a guide, has its own hazards.

In studies of UDOR conducted at twenty programs over a two-year period, there was one death; TUDOR, in turn, is associated with blood in the urine, postoperative pain, bladder and kidney infections and, in some cases, with a recurrence of pelvic inflammatory disease. Puncture of the blood vessels and/or bowel is rare, but reported.

Some risks of inducing ovulation with fertility drugs include enlargement of the ovaries (hypertrophy), ovarian cysts, irregular period after treatment ends, and a set of PMS-like symptoms that can include emotional instability, breast tenderness, and hot flashes. Clomiphene citrate (Chlomid or Serophene) is actually an antiestrogen that destroys fertile mucus in some cases, so yet another drug is given to replace estrogen.

Pergonal or human menopausal gonadotropin (HMG), a gonad stimulating hormone, is an expensive mixture of FSH (follicle stimulating hormone) and LH (luteinizing hormone) given in a very stressful regimen of daily injections. Progesterone injections and human chorionic gonadotropin used by some infertility specialists for "luteal phase support" have not been proven to increase pregnancy success in randomized controlled trials.

Bromocriptine (Parlodel) is not used to stimulate the ovaries, but to lower excess prolactin (a hormone that stimulates lactation) levels that can suppress ovulation. The side effects of Parlodel include low blood pressure, dizziness, and headache, among many others. Parlodel is, unfortunately, used extensively in obstetrics to suppress lactation. For more information, please consult the *Birth Journal* and read "Hormonal Problems and Their Treatment" by Carla Harkness in *The Infertility Book* (see recommended readings).

With ovulation induction, fertility drugs (clomiphene citrate and Pergonal) force the ovaries to ripen multiple follicles, not just one egg. The process of superovulation in combination with the multiple transfer of embryos to increase IVF/ET success results in a significantly higher rate of pregnancy with multiples (20 percent twins, higher with Pergonal; 3 percent triplets), and pregnancy and birth with multiples are associated with known perinatal health hazards, including prematurity.

In addition to pressures associated with the burden of caring for more than one infant at a time, these problems are addressed by Frances V. Price in "The Risk of High Multiparty with IVF/ET" in *Birth*, Fall 1988.

There also is the ethical question of what to do with extra embryos that are currently frozen and stored in nitrous oxide. Already, bizarre legal disputes have risen over ownership of the embryo after divorce, and the issue of embryo experimentation is a concern to feminists and fundamentalists alike.

In her work entitled "In Vitro Fertilization: Reflections on the State of the Art" (*Birth: Issues in Perinatal Care and Education*, Fall 1988), Dr. Helen B. Holmes described the larger number of birth defects reported in a new Australian study of 1697 IVF births: 6.7 times the expected occurrence of transposition of the great vessels (heart defect); 5 times as many cases of spina bifida (open spinal cord); and 1.3 times more cases of hypospadias (abnormal opening in the urethra). Equally ominous is Holmes's statement that it is reasonable to speculate "that women treated with fertility drugs, especially repeatedly, will be at risk for endometrial, cervical, ovarian, and breast cancer for two to three decades."

As if this were not enough, the long-term effect of ultrasound on an ovum, embryo, and fetus is still unknown. Yet, in the IVF/ET process, ultrasound is used frequently to visualize the interior of the woman's body and to track follicular growth. Everyone agrees that exposure to *non-ionizing* radiation with ultrasound is safer than receiving *ionizing* radiation with X-ray. However, there are troubling reports in animal studies, and the general consensus in obstetrics is to use the technology only when medically indicated; unfortunately, however, this recommendation has been largely ignored.

At a 1989 symposium entitled "Innovations in Perinatal Care: Assessing Benefits and Risks," Dr. Kenneth J. W. Taylore recommended that radiologists and ultrasound technicians use the following safety measures: equipment with high resolution (to get a clear picture) and the lowest possible dose; know the dose (technicians, even physicians, do not always know the dose put out by their machines); better training; more research; and, of interest to IVF/ET candidates, share research findings with patients so they can make an informed choice about accepting or rejecting ultrasound for diagnosis or treatment.

In Vitro Fertilization/Embryo Transfer (IVF/ET)

IVF is a biologically and technically complicated procedure which is still new and experimental. It is available to women whose ovaries and uterus appear to function normally, but whose fallopian tubes are blocked and do not function properly so the egg cannot get to the uterus. Under present regulations in the U.S., women must also be married.

About 600,000 American women are in this situation but, at present, only very few centers offer the procedure. Though IVF costs between 2,500 and 4,000 dollars, plus the medical expenses associated with pregnancy and birth, thousands of women are waiting to be screened to determine whether or not they meet the clinics' criteria.

In vitro is Latin for "in glass." In in vitro fertilization, the technical feat is to extract a ripe egg from the ovary, fertilize it with sperm in a glass dish, and get the embryo back into the womb. The first successful in vitro fertilization and subsequent implantation was achieved in England in November 1977 and resulted in the birth of Louise Brown. Since then, babies conceived in vitro have been born in different parts of the world and, at this writing, several hundred women are carrying fetuses conceived by IVF.

Different physicians and clinics are developing their own modifications, but the procedure involves these steps:

A woman who wants to try IVF first undergoes a battery of screening procedures, which often include surgery to make her ovaries accessible for collecting eggs. The practitioner must collect the egg just before it would normally be released. (Human eggs are so small that they are hard to find once they've left the follicle.) To pinpoint the precise time when a follicle will release an egg, the practitioner examines the ovaries with ultrasound and measures hormone levels. (Physicians now use ultrasound as though they know it is safe and assure pregnant women of its safety, but one cannot yet be sure. It took several decades before the risks of X-rays were obvious. We must worry about this, especially when it's a question of irradiating our ovaries or early embryos with ultrasound, because their cells divide frequently and dividing cells tend to be especially sensitive to all forms of radiation.) To have more control of the timing of ovulation, most physicians now administer hormones called gonadotropins. Unfortunately, gonadotropins somewhat increase the chances that the eggs will have chromosomal abnormalities, such as the chromosome duplication responsible for Down's syndrome. They also induce several eggs to mature at the same time, something that ordinarily happens only rarely.

The physician then collects ripe eggs from the ovary by a surgical procedure known as laparoscopy, which at present is done under general anesthesia. During the laparoscopy, s/he punctures the follicle(s) and draws out the egg(s) by gentle suction. (The image the surgeon sees with the laparoscope can be projected onto a screen so that the entire operating team can see it.) S/he places the egg in a clean, sterilized dish containing a nutrient solution and mixes it with a sample of newly ejaculated sperm. The covered dish is placed in an incubator at normal body temperature and examined from time to time under a microscope.

If all goes well, one of the 20,000 or so sperm in the sample will enter the egg, the egg and sperm nuclei (the organelles where the chromosomes are) will fuse and, within a few hours, the fertilized egg will divide first into two cells, then four, and so on. The cells remain attached to each other and form the early embryo.

Some clinics transfer the embryo into the womb at the two-cell stage; others wait until it has four or six cells. If the cells look normal under the microscope, one or two embryos are introduced into the mother's womb, so that one or both can attach and develop further. At this time, no one knows how to make a human embryo survive outside the womb past these earliest stages.

In order for the physician to transfer an embryo into the womb, the woman lies on her back with her knees up, as she would for a cervical exam, on a table that is sometimes tilted about twenty degrees head down. Her vagina and cervix are swabbed with sterile salt solution, and the physician sucks the embryo and a drop of the solution in which it has been growing into a tube that is the width of a thin straw; then s/he inserts this tube into the womb through the vagina and cervix. By means of gentle positive pressure, the embryo in its drop of fluid is expelled into the womb, and the tube is slowly pulled out. This takes only a few minutes and is done without anesthesia.

At this point, everyone waits to see whether the embryo will implant—the step that most often fails during the entire procedure. Even with natural fertilizations, probably only about one in four embryos implants properly and the rest are lost. At this time with IVF, chances are more likely one in ten.

If the embryo doesn't implant, the entire procedure, including the laparoscopy, must be repeated.

Once we decide to try IVF, many of us are prepared to come back if we don't become pregnant the first time, though clinics usually limit the number of times a woman can try. To avoid the need for repeated anesthesia and surgery, physicians are giving women so-called "fertility drugs," which make several eggs mature simultaneously (gonadotropin hormones—see above). They can then collect several eggs during one laparoscopy and fertilize them all in vitro. Some physicians then transfer two (or more) embryos into the womb, hoping that at least one will implant. Of course, if both implant, you can end up with twins, and multiple pregnancies sometimes involve increased health risks for mothers and babies. Others also freeze a few for storage and possible later insertion if the first implantation doesn't succeed, but so far, physicians have had little or no luck getting frozen and thawed embryos to implant. At present, no one knows the risks of this procedure.

The physicians who use IVF believe that the risks are negligible. They argue that if an egg or embryo is damaged, it simply won't develop, but we won't know whether that's true until thousands of babies conceived in vitro have had a chance to grow up. This is why some critics of IVF, as of other reproductive technologies, have said that in this procedure, women and their babies become guinea pigs.

And what of the ethical, legal, and emotional issues? A procedure that requires this much technical expertise is completely under professional control. We and our partners will never have much say about where or how we want it done. Because the pregnancies are so precious (emotionally, technically, and economically), couples are under pressure to manage the prenatal period and birth just as the physicians order. Many women who have IVF are having cesareans, and when Ms. Brown was expecting

Louise, she even had to agree in writing that she would have an abortion if Dr. Steptoe and Edwards thought she should!

> *As thousands of women try to enroll in IVF programs, we must question why it is that many of us gladly accept painful medical interventions and unknown health risks in order to bear a child. We must look at the socialization we undergo as women which makes childbearing seem more important than our own health and well-being. We mustn't feel pressured by the fact that this technology now is available. There is nothing wrong with us as women if we decide not to become involved with complicated, expensive, and experimental procedures whose risks cannot be known with certainty for a long time.*
>
> *Clearly, the procedure is sufficiently expensive, complex, and of such uncertain outcome that it can serve relatively few of us. Meanwhile, many of us will risk invasive exploratory procedures and repeated attempts at IVF only to end up disappointed. IVF is yet another example of the way the medical profession develops high-technology "solutions" to preventable problems instead of stressing simple preventive measures that could serve many more of us. Most of us who end up wanting IVF would not need it if we had known earlier about possible* preventable *long-term effects of untreated or mistreated pelvic inflammatory and sexually transmitted disease, and about risks from I.U.D.s and other birth control methods that physicians often urge on us.*

From *The New Our Bodies, Ourselves*

Thoughts on IVF/ET

Endometriosis and blocked fallopian tubes are the problems most likely to lead women to consider in vitro fertilization (IVF).

If opting for IVF, the reader needs to know her rights as a hospitalized patient and may even wish to consider alternatives, such as donor insemination and adoption.

To best understand how IVF/ET works, the reader needs to become familiar with its seven essential steps.

Step 1. The patients are selected. Married couples or couples in a committed heterosexual relationship, who meet physical and psychological eligibility criteria are chosen and, if they can pay the 6,000 to 8,000 dollar tab for each IVF/ET attempt, they are placed on a waiting list (some clinics ask for a commitment of four attempts). In terms of physical health, the woman usually must be thirty-five years of age or younger, of average weight, and have at least one functioning ovary.

If the partner's sperm is to be used for IVF, he must pass a semen evaluation.

Subsequent steps proceed *only* if the first step is successful; otherwise, the attempt—referred to as a "stimulation cycle"—is cancelled. If the couple opts to continue, the process must begin anew.

Step 2. This is a chemical induction of ovulation. Under the influence of fertility drugs, follicular growth is stimulated and then monitored by ultrasound. Estrogen and LH concentrations are evaluated through daily blood and urine tests. If the leading follicle develops to the proper size, additional hormones to trigger ovulation are given.

Step 3. Retrieval of the eggs is timed to harvest the eggs surgically before ovulation takes place. If timing is off, the attempt is cancelled; otherwise, the surgeon aspirates three to twelve eggs through a laparoscope (an in-hospital procedure done under general anesthetic) or uses one of the newer ultrasonic procedures (UDOR—ultrasonically directed oocyte retrieval or UGA—ultrasonically guided aspiration, and TUDOR—transvaginal UDOR) to locate and harvest the eggs through the vagina, bladder, or abdomen. These are outpatient procedures.

Step 4. At this step, the man produces semen by masturbating. His sperm is then "washed" and otherwise treated to bring the strongest sperm to the top of the sample.

Step 5. At this step, fertilization and cleavage, eggs and sperm are incubated. If fertilization occurs and embryonic development begins within the next two days, the doctor proceeds to the next step.

Step 6. Transfer of the embryo. Up to four embryos are inserted into the woman's uterus (woman awake, usually in knee-chest position). Gamete intra-fallopian transfer (GIFT) is an alternate procedure for women with at least one healthy fallopian tube. GIFT combines steps 3, 4, 5, and 6 to plant the newly retrieved eggs and sperm directly into the fallopian tubes where, hopefully, fertilization will take place.

Step 7. Chemical implantation. When successful, this procedure results in a "chemical pregnancy." Unfortunately, the spontaneous abortion rate is over 50 percent and, according to Helen B. Holmes, writing in "In Vitro Fertilization: Reflections on the State of the Art," published in *Birth: Issues in Perinatal Care and Education*, Fall 1988, ectopic pregnancies and preterm births are higher than they are in the general population. In 1988, Holmes reported on the risks of infertility diagnosis and treatment to the U.S. Congress Office of Technology Assessment. Her summary provided one resource for this discussion.

Holmes said the actual birth rate with IVF/ET is less than 10 percent. Some IVF/ET programs, however, claim a success rate of 20 percent by counting the number of chemical pregnancies as opposed to realistic figures based on live births.

Be sure to ask for solid statistics on take-home babies, not on "probable" births.

IVF/ET is at best a very complex, uncertain process. Despite its many rigors, however, the one in nine or ten successful couples express great appreciation for the technology. If the reader is interested, she should read the Holmes article (the public library can get a reprint) and the following books: Menning's *Infertility: A Guide for the Childless Couple*; Perloe and Christie's *Miracle Babies*, and Harkness' *The Infertility Book: A Comprehensive Medical and Emotional Guide* (see Recommended Readings).

The reader will also want to join RESOLVE, an organization that will put her in touch with a support group and furnish an IVF clinic list along with their waiting times. RESOLVE also has updated information about health insurance and infertility treatment.

Margot Edwards; R.N., M.A.

Is It Worth It? I Just Don't Know

This piece is based on a discussion between Anne Stuart, an Australian woman, and Renate Klein. Anne Stuart is a pseudonym. She feels that being critical of the IVF program in public could jeopardize her chances of continuing on the program.

I've been through three IVF cycles: two full ones and one with frozen embryos. In each case, I had a successful embryo transfer. No one knows why it didn't work. I still have three frozen embryos in storage, and if the next frozen cycle isn't successful, I don't know if I will continue with the program.

In retrospect, I wonder why I didn't realize that I had a fertility problem earlier. But I didn't and it came as a shock when I found out that I was infertile. In fact, when I didn't become pregnant I assumed my husband was having problems.

I'd had a Copper Seven I.U.D. inserted when I was nineteen. I thought it was a responsible act of contraception. Right from the beginning, the I.U.D. was very painful and I had a lot of bleeding. I lost weight rapidly, and I was tired and listless. So I asked my doctor to remove it, but he told me my problems would settle down. I also told him that I found sexual intercourse very painful. He put my complaints down to emotional problems and referred me to a psychiatrist. The psychiatrist told me that there was nothing wrong with me, but a year later I still hadn't convinced my doctor to remove the I.U.D. I changed doctors and my new doctor removed it on my first visit. He started treating me for thrush and mentioned that he suspected that my womb may have been ruptured by the I.U.D.

I went from one doctor to another trying to find a cure for constant vaginal infections and pains in my sides. Meanwhile, my tubes were becoming badly infected, and I was starting to believe that I was neurotic.

I stopped taking the Pill when I was twenty-five. Two years later I still hadn't become pregnant. This didn't worry me at first, but after two years my husband and I started having tests. Despite my medcial history, I still didn't think that I had a fertility problem—I assumed it was my husband.

I had blood tests to see if I was ovulating and my husband had a sperm count done. Then, my tubes were injected with dye to see if they were blocked. They must have been in a very bad way because none of the dye went through.

I finally had a laparoscopy, which showed that my tubes were completely blocked from years of infection. Though my gynecologist wouldn't openly support my theory that it was caused by the I.U.D., he didn't discount it either.

I feel that there is stigma attached to the word "infection." The doctors gave me the impression that they suspected my constant infections were related to sexual promiscuity. I had to undergo all sorts of tests, including tests for AIDS, chlamydia, and venereal diseases. The results of all of these tests were negative, but my infertility is still described in my doctor's medical notes as pelvic inflammatory disease (which, to my knowledge, is nearly always associated with chlamydia). Also, coming from a small town, where everyone knows everyone else, it was quite embarrassing to go to pathology for a barrage of tests which are linked to social diseases.

I almost felt vindicated when my first laparoscopy showed that I did have a physical problem. Although I was very disappointed, it proved that I wasn't merely neurotic.

I still wasn't having a very good run with doctors, though. When I came out of the anesthetic, my gynecologist wandered over to my bed and said in front of the other patients in my ward, "It doesn't look like there's much chance there. I think I'd better send you to Professor X." This was totally unexpected, yet I couldn't even show any grief over the news because I was surrounded by three other patients recovering from wisdom-teeth operations.

So Professor X performed microsurgery on my fallopian tubes. The right tube was beyond repair and he removed it altogether. He did his best to repair the left one. He didn't give me any details about the consequences of the operation, but I found out through my own research that I would be more likely to have an ectopic pregnancy.

I was glad that I had found this out because two years later I actually had an ectopic pregnancy. As soon as I realized I was pregnant, I felt that there was something wrong. I had a dull ache in my left side, but again I had to convince my gynecologist that I wasn't neurotic. I started bleeding, but his receptionist wouldn't let me speak to him. In the end, I rang my G.P. and asked him to contact the gynecologist on my behalf. He convinced my gynecologist to see me, and I had to undergo emergency surgery that same afternoon.

After I came back from surgery, my gynecologist, true to form, said, "It was really bad luck about that pregnancy: the fetus was only a quarter of a centimeter away from the uterus." This really upset me. It would have been better if he'd said nothing. I changed gynecologists after that.

I waited twelve months to get on the IVF program's waiting list, and then it took me another twelve months before I started the treatment. It seemed that every month another obstacle would be placed in my way. My husband would need another sperm count, or I would need an AIDS test, or I'd be waiting on the phone for so long to get through to the infertility center, that that day's quota of women would be filled. Their regulations seemed to change from month to month, but nobody told me what was going on.

Two years after placing my name on the waiting list, I finally had my first treatment. The whole procedure was very stressful, both from a physical and emotional point of view. I'd get up at 5 a.m. to drive to Melbourne for HMG injections and blood tests. I also had to take Clomid tablets twice a day for the first five days. As my ovulation time got closer, I had blood tests in the evening. Just prior to the egg pickup I was given an HCG injection.

When I had to have blood tests done in the evening, I'd sometimes do the one hour drive to Melbourne after work and stay overnight. Then I'd drive back to work after my morning blood test. The hospital to which the infertility clinic is attached won't treat outpatients anymore, so now I have to have the evening test done at my local hospital and take it with me in the morning.

I had two vaginal ultrasounds to check on the progress of my eggs. I still have visions of a technician telling me to relax while he inserts an instrument that looks like a giant dildo into my vagina. It's not supposed to hurt if it's done properly, but I found it very uncomfortable.

The ultrasound was also used to collect the eggs during the pickup. Eight eggs were collected and six were fertilized—three were transferred and the other three were frozen. My first treatment took place during the nurses' strike, and for some reason operations could only take place after 6 p.m. I was the only one left in my ward who actually got to the stage of having a pickup and transfer. In several instances, women ovulated before their operation could be scheduled.

I was very nervous the first time I had an embryo transfer. My cervix was scraped and a long, think catheter was inserted into my vagina, and the eggs were released into it. It wasn't really painful, but it felt like a very strong cramp.

I wasn't supposed to move for at least half an hour after the transfer, but after lying in the recovery room for ten minutes, I was wheeled down the corridor at top speed and transferred to a bed. The bed was then pushed back against the wall. I was aware that I had to lie still until my cervix had closed and that this probably would have happened within the first ten minutes after the transfer. But I feel that my rapid trip from the recovery room to the ward couldn't have helped the situation.

I went home and took things quietly, but five days before my period was due, I started to bleed. I was quite upset that the treatment hadn't been successful and yet I was surprised that I *was* so upset because I hadn't really expected it to work the first time.

My husband was quite supportive, but I knew he was disappointed. We really didn't discuss the issue. I know that it's better to discuss these things, but I didn't want to think about it.

We had to pay a 250 dollar storage fee for the frozen embryos. I couldn't claim any of this on my health insurance. In fact my three IVF attempts have cost us 10,000 (Australian) dollars over and above what we could claim on our health insurance, and the costs are increasing all the time. There is a surcharge on IVF consultancy fees, and I can't even claim for Clomid tablets anymore.

Four months after my first treatment, I tried a frozen cycle. The three eggs were defrosted, but only one was suitable for transfer. I really hadn't expected the frozen cycle to work because I knew that the success rate was very low, so I wasn't very disappointed when I got my period.

On my last full cycle, six eggs were collected—three were frozen and three transferred. I was more optimistic this time because I had lasted right up to the due date of my period without bleeding. I was disappointed when my period arrived because I thought I had passed the critical stage. I still don't know why it didn't work. In hindsight, I wonder if they were experimenting on me, because on the form I received specifying the number of eggs that were frozen, I noticed that two had been frozen at the 4-cell stage, but one had been frozen at the 5-cell stage. If the embryos that had been transferred were also at the 5-cell stage, I don't think a pregnancy would have been possible.

Apart from the fact that I have never achieved a pregnancy on the IVF program, my treatment has always gone like clockwork. After the last treatment was again unsuccessful, I didn't bother to pay a visit to Professor X, although I've since found out that this is compulsory. I resent paying fifty dollars to be told that he doesn't know why the treatment isn't working.

The infertility center has now introduced a system where patients must have a consultation with an IVF doctor when they come in for their blood tests each morning. This means that I have to pay for a consultation every day while I'm on an IVF cycle, even though the doctor just checks my hormone levels on a chart and tells me to come back the next day. Last time, even when my own doctor, Professor X, was the consulting physician, I had to remind him that I was due for an egg pickup. He was very vague. He forgot to tell one of the women who started with me that she needed an ultrasound. By the time she had one, it was too late. She'd already ovulated.

I think that Professor X is more interested in the research side of IVF than its humanitarian aspects. I suppose for a lot of the people on the IVF team, the procedures have become routine. This was really brought home to me when I had my last embryo transfer. The doctor who did the transfer didn't acknowledge my presence. He spoke to the sister standing next to me but gave no indication that I was a participant in the procedure. When he had finished, I was wheeled out and he didn't even look up.

One of the most frustrating aspects of the program is the lack of information. As soon as my name was put on the IVF waiting list I started to research the program. Professor X is the co-author of a book on in vitro fertilization, which gave me some basic information. But I wanted to know why it was essential that I take hormones to superovulate. I know that I won't produce as many eggs naturally, but they may be of a better quality without chemical interference. I also wonder how my body could be physically able to accept an embryo after my hormone balance has been chemically altered so drastically. After all, this is not the way a woman's body would normally function if she were pregnant. One of my major concerns is the long-term effect of the drugs I am using, both on myself and on my child if I were to become pregnant.

I don't have a medical background, but I don't think that these are such strange questions. I feel that my questions have been played down. I have been told that there will be no long-term problems, but I still haven't received any satisfactory answers. This is one of the reasons I have long breaks between treatments, so my body has time to recover. After each full cycle you must have a three month break, but I don't know if this is long enough. One woman I spoke to had had eight treatments in a row and she was a nervous wreck. I don't know whether she was suffering from the normal stresses associated with the program, but I'm sure that the large doses of hormones wouldn't have helped.

I'm also worried about the IVF's higher than usual rate of abnormalities. One woman I met had had triplets through the program. Two of her children were fine, but the third had spina bifida. I also know of a woman who had developed cancer of the womb after taking clomiphene citrate. She wasn't on the IVF program, but she was taking it as a fertility stimulant.

Perhaps I'm over-sensitive, but I get the impression that I have no right to question the IVF procedures or to ask the staff to simplify any of the routines for my benefit. For example, many of the tests which my husband and I have had to undergo could have been done in our own town. But this is not acceptable to the infertility center. So we have to take time off work and spend an hour driving to Melbourne, sometimes for the sake of a ten-minute procedure. I must admit that I haven't been very assertive about my rights because I feel that if I were known to be a troublemaker it could jeopardize my chances to continue on the program.

My greatest frustration in being involved with the IVF program is the lack of information available to me. It also entails a great deal of stress—physically, emotionally and financially. It's meant that my whole life—my work, my study, and my marriage—is at a standstill until I become pregnant or give it up.

Having children is important to me, but I still feel that I can lead a fulfilling life without being a mother, but being childless has really affected my husband. He doesn't discuss it very often, but I know that to him, a marriage is not complete without children. I've even thought about being altruistic and giving him a divorce so he can find someone who can give him a child before it's too late. But I guess I'm too selfish to really do that. So, for as long as I'm married, I'll probably never accept that we'll be childless.

We haven't seriously considered adoption, mainly because the adoption lists in Australia aren't even open and even if they were, by the time we reached the top of the list, we'd be too old to qualify. Also, it is very important to my husband that he has his own, genetic child.

If my husband and I were to split up, I wouldn't persevere with the program. I am going through this because I've put ten years into our relationship, but if I had another partner, he would just have to accept that I can't have children.

When we were first married, we both had certain expectations, one being that eventually we would have children. My infertility has changed many of our expectations. Financially, we're better off than if we had had children, and I've had to really think about my career, whereas with a family I may not have been able to make certain career choices—I may have just stopped working and stayed at home. It has also meant that I've been able to take on a more independent role than I would have done with family commitments. Socially, we're in limbo— we just don't fit in. Of course we have friends, both single and married, but none of them can really understand our situation.

Perhaps I should have joined the IVF Friends, but I really feel that my infertility is a personal problem. Part of the reason for this is that I didn't want it to dominate my life, but I also think that, deep down, I'm ashamed of my inability to produce a child, especially when it seems so easy for other women. I've been aware that I am infertile for six years, and I still find it difficult to discuss it openly.

Being infertile has forced me to take control of my own life. I can't just drift along and let things take their course. I have to make decisions—about my career, about my marriage, and about children. Superficially, the IVF program offers me a simple choice—the chance to stay on the program and perhaps have a child, or the chance to stop and accept my infertility. But my decision is not so clear cut—the stress, the constant uncertainty, my fear of the treatment's long-term effects, and the lack of control that I have over the treatment, make me wonder if I would have been better off not having to make a decision.

Is it worth it? I just don't know.

He Called Me Number 27

Inge M. (thirty-two), a full-time homemaker from West Germany with two adopted children, went through IVF in 1982. The procedure was not successful. The interview was conducted and edited by Ute Winkler (twenty-nine), in 1987. Inge's husband Peter (twenty-six) was present during the interview.

Ute: Could you please begin by telling me how you came to IVF?

Inge: We got married in 1979 and wanted children as soon as possible. We waited for two years and then it did not work. A laparoscopic examination showed that my fallopian tubes were completely blocked and full of adhesions and scar tissue. Microsurgery would have been possible, and we were told that the chances for success were about 5 percent, but my gynecologist advised against such an operation. So, at that stage there were three options: no children at all (but that, of course, was not offered as an option); IVF (a procedure which is called "extracorporal"); or adoption.

Upon hearing this, I went into a deep depression. Then, we started two things at once: I made an appointment with Professor T in X, and at the same time, we put our names down for adoption with the Youth Welfare Department.

Ute: You contacted Professor T yourselves?

Inge: Yes. At first we were told that there was a waiting list of four to five years; that, too, was a reason for my depression. The Youth Welfare Department had also given us a waiting time of four to five years, the same as Professor T. But then we got a phone call from T informing us that I was going to be accepted into his program immediately. I think my age was very important, and also the fact that I was physically fit and psychologically balanced, except for those depressions. I was ovulating and my hormones seemed O.K. It is very important to be fit and well for IVF. If one is already totally out of order, there is little chance of success. We were then asked to send in my temperature charts.

Ute: Up to that time you had never been in X and you had never spoken to Professor T? All you had done was to send him your case history, which you got from your gynecologist?

Inge: Yes. I sent all my surgery reports and everything else. Next we were asked to come for an examination to make sure that the reports we had sent were correct. This preliminary examination was done by a biologist. He said that everything was O.K. and that my treatment was to start in September. He gave me a prescription and I was to swallow hormones—Dynerik tablets they were—for three to four days beginning five days after my period. I had terrible reactions to them! Well, I took these tablets for awhile and then we went to X. We took a room in a hotel, and I had to go to the clinic every day for a blood test to check my hormone levels. Every day I had an ultrasound to monitor the development of my ovaries. I am very regular, as I know that I'll get my period every twenty-sixth day in the afternoon. It was quite clear to me why they were so keen to have me on the program. The hormones they gave me speeded the whole procedure up, but in my case, they were able to calculate everything very well in advance.

The ultrasounds were agony. One has to drink a lot of water so as to have a full bladder, because only in this way are the ovaries visible. There we sat, about seven or nine women. At first we could not stand each other. We felt like enemies. We did not speak to each other, just exchanged hostile glances, because each of us wanted to be the first. Each expected to be the one who was successful. None wanted one of the others to start egg collection before her. I knew that I would be one of the first because of my regular twenty-six-day cycle.

Well, after a while we got to know each other, and things were less tense. Once the women started to speak about themselves, the things that came out really required strong nerves. I can understand that none of the doctors want to have anything to do with their private lives. If they did, they probably could not do their jobs. Professor T was rather cold.

Ute: But in public he acts as if he were a great benefactor.

Inge: Until he gets his people! Maybe he has improved since I knew him four years ago. I also think that he wants to advertise his cause. One of the problems is that many of the women who sit in his waiting room have already reached the upper age limit. People who try for a test-tube baby are usually desperate. Mostly, they are no longer young women. Between twenty-five and thirty one can say, well, I've still got time, I can try this or that. But if nothing happens at thirty-eight, thirty-nine, or forty, then this is their last chance, because at their age they are also too old for adoption. So there are only the Professor T's, because by then all the other medical possibilities have been exhausted. It's the last chance, and if it fails, a whole mountain of hopes and dreams comes tumbling down.

So there we were—women drinking water and none of us dared to go to the toilet. Now, say the appointment was at 9 a.m. Ten women come in at 9 a.m. with bladders so full you think they're going to burst any minute. But the doctor only appears at 10:30. Try yourself to wait for an hour-and-a-half with a full bladder; one feels like exploding! I remember how one of the women could not control herself any longer. She went to the toilet and passed a little water. Unfortunately, she was called in immediately after. You should have heard how they shouted at her in front of everybody: "You are just sitting here with nothing else to do the whole day and you can't even control yourself," etc., etc. And these women are thirty-five to forty years old. They really should not have to put up with this kind of treatment.

Finally, after all those daily ultrasound checkups, we were all called together and each woman was informed how far she had come in her monthly cycle. One woman was told that she had been ovulating the previous day. She should try again in two months' time.

Ute: So you are saying that you had a meeting where each woman's cycle was publicly discussed?

Inge: Yes. Every woman's cycle was public knowledge. So we all sat there and Professor T called me Number Twenty-Seven. I must have looked rather puzzled, so he quickly added my name. I think he mixed us up with his numbers. We all looked around and thought what was it that we didn't understand this time? And we were all so nervous. I don't care how he identifies me in his paperwork, but in public he has no right to address me as a number.

Well, I was to be done the next day. I had to go to the hospital at 3 a.m. and the nurse on night duty gave me the hormone injection. Then back to the hotel and on the next day I was admitted to the clinic. This was the time when the eggs had to be collected within twelve hours, that is to say as late as possible, but not too late, because the egg membrane could break and then the egg would be lost. To catch an egg just before ovulation, that is T's great specialty. He is really good at that. I suppose that's why IVF requires a cool scientist, not somebody who messes around with feelings.

Ute: He must be prepared to take risks. I mean he must postpone the moment as long as possible without, however, missing it.

Inge: Yes, that's right. But with many women he *did* miss the moment. These women can then only try again in two to three months. Many of them cried. One woman had noticed her ovulation during the night, but the doctor said that was not possible. They just did not believe her. But at the ultrasound they discovered it too, and the woman was sent home in tears.

Ute: So what happened next, once you were admitted to the hospital?

Inge: First, I had another blood test to check the hormone levels and another ultrasound. But this time it was different. The bladder had to be full again, but because of the general anesthetic that was to follow for egg collection, it could not be filled via the stomach. So they put me on a drip with a sugar solution. Normally they allow two hours for the bladder to be filled up, but they were late putting me on the drip so they hurried it up—it took only half an hour. My arm got terribly cold!

Once on the drip one cannot walk any more, and so they took me upstairs to the ultrasound in a wheelchair.

The room adjacent to the ultrasound was again full of women I had met before. They all waited for T or his assistants. It was clear to them now that I was the first to be done, and they were all curious to see how I would do. But this time there was neither envy nor animosity, only interest and tension. The ultrasound went well and the doctors kept saying to me "look here" and "look there," but I could not see a thing. Then I was taken out of the ultrasound room and the women outside clapped their hands and said, "Quick now, downstairs to the theater!" That was a great demonstration of solidarity. The rivalry was only in the beginning when everyone wanted to be the first.

So I was taken to the theater and they gave me an injection. This made me very anxious and frightened. They also put me on the heart machine, but that guy, that T, just would not appear—it was disgusting. Here I was, semi-conscious and they left me completely alone in the room. Finally, I screamed that somebody should come and stay with me. I could not bear to be left alone with all those machines. Because of the monitor, I felt that my heart was somewhere in the room, and it went faster and faster. But nobody came and I got into a total panic. So I said that I was going to leave, that I could not cope, that I wanted to get out. I would have torn off all those tubes, but at that moment, T arrived.

It is no good if a patient is in a panic because of the anesthetic. The anesthetist told T that I had gone crazy. And T said: "What's the matter with her? I am here!" And he signalled to them to put me out. I had had to wait for him for an hour-and-a-half, and my feet had gone very cold. It was a very long hour because I was terrified that I could have ovulated. I was lying on the operating table and fantasized that the eggs had jumped ou,t and that T would open me up and find that the eggs had gone. Then he could have told me any old story.

But luckily everything went well, just as he had expected. He found two egg cells and one of them began to divide. They usually find two to three egg cells, never just one. Often there are many more, but they don't like that very much because every egg that divides has to be put back. That is because of the law or ethical principles, I think. In any case, that is what they told us. Everything that is taken out and that divides has to be transferred to the woman's womb.

Ute: Would you have preferred it if they had found more egg cells?

Inge: I would not have liked it, for instance, if they had taken six egg cells which all developed. Nobody wants that much good luck! Just imagine what it would be like to get six children all at once. Twins could have been all right, but six! And usually one or more babies from multiple births have health problems—that's another risk one doesn't want.

Well, they took me back to the ward, and I had to rest for forty-eight hours. Then they transferred the one egg cell which had divided. That too was quite an impossible business, though not from a medical point of view. Peter wanted to be present at the transfer. He wanted to come with me in that room where the gynecological chair stood. In any case, he was the father, or would have been, but they absolutely refused and the way they did it was anything but tactful. They looked at him as if to say, "Who do you think you are?" T was terrible. So cold. In the end, the room was crowded with people who were allowed to watch: a professor from Australia, a student, three female assistants, and two nurses. People everywhere, but there was no room for Peter. Then they started talking as if I wasn't there. During the whole procedure, T never said anything nice or encouraging to me. I had the feeling that he never noticed that I was even there. Not that I had expected much in the way of empathy, but T did not look me in the face once. I heard him saying, "Oh look, how beautiful!" But it was always the others who were asked to look how beautiful I was down there. How would I know what was so beautiful! " And now we insert the probe . . ." and this and that. But of course I could not see anything as I was lying on my back. I found the whole procedure really inhuman. If only they would do it in a more humane way! I am sure they would be more successful. From a psychological point of view, the whole business is so complicated and hard to take that one just has to reject it, both from a rational and from an emotional point of view. It is just so artificial; so alienating . . . I could only go through with it because one of the nurses was just so totally nice.

Another thing was that they had put us in the maternity ward. It didn't matter much to me, but for other women it was just the last straw, it really finished them off. Our nice nurse always saw to it that we were reasonably happy and comfortable and she laughed and joked with us. We used to call T "God Almighty." Well he was, wasn't he? So we used to say, "Here comes God Almighty . . . ."

Later, when T took over a clinic closer to where we live, he wrote to us and asked if we wanted to try again, especially since I had such a good cycle, and it would be so handy for us now. . . After the laparoscopy (for egg collection), T had also advised us to have microsurgery. "It wouldn't be so bad . . . ." he said. My own gynecologist, however, suggested, "Do whatever you like, but they are all researchers and scientists, they need guinea pigs, the microsurgeons included. They need people on whom they can practice."

If I had become pregnant, I don't know whether I would have told T about it at all. Under no circumstances would I have wanted him for the birth; the whole procedure, the things I lived through, the other women and their sufferings, and the way they were treated. At twenty-seven it is probably easier to cope with these things than at forty!

Ute: I cannot understand why T does not take the women seriously, particularly when he must know that the success of the transfer of the fertilized egg has a lot to do with how the woman feels.

Inge: T believes he can trick the psyche. That's the whole point. Can the psyche be tricked or can't it? I don't believe it is possible. I found the whole thing repulsive. One really has to believe it; and perhaps if one doesn't see any other way, it might work. . . .

Ute: Were you very disappointed when it did not work for you?

Inge: I didn't really believe in it ever! Perhaps this is why it did not work. The disappointment was really like the other monthly disappointments when, again, it had not worked. But in the first few months afterward, it was very hard for us to speak about it because of our hurt feelings about how we had been treated. But the more time passes, the better I can cope. I don't think I would do it again. We would very much like a third child, and it is hard to make up one's mind. I would love to be able to decide for myself whether I'll have a third child or not. I think that I have a right to have ten children, but unfortunately there is this problem . . . sometimes I wonder if we should try again . . . but then we would again be dependent on some professor who would torture us in the same way, or even more, because there would be the whole medical procedure again.

Ute: Is it important for both of you to have your own biological child?

Inge: When the gynecologist told me that I could not have any children of my own, it was terrible to think that I could never have a child around me of whom I could say, "Look, it is just like me." Childlessness causes suffering, sometimes it hurts, sometimes it doesn't. I have times when I cry a lot. This will always be so—we will always have our ups and downs. That's quite normal, one is always mourning for something that might have been. Sometimes I don't feel it for a year, and I think all is well. And then, suddenly, it is there again. It can be caused by anything, a birthday, a certain smell, anything that reminds me of a child.

Ute: Just to return to T once again. Were you told about risks and success rates? Or how the whole IVF procedure is done, in detail?

Inge: Not much. I understood things most of the time and I asked questions. I can look after myself reasonably well, but there was a woman from another country who didn't understand a thing of what was happening to her. Her husband was the same. A young doctor, whose job it was to explain everything to that couple, noticed that they had a language problem, but he was not prepared to spend more time with them. With the woman they could do as they pleased, as we were in the clinic. But the husband had to understand when he had to bring in his sperm, or else the whole procedure would have been useless. We were not really informed about what would happen. They told us very briefly about the whole physiological procedure. The ethics of the whole thing was not discussed.

Ute: Did they tell you about the success rates?

Inge: At the time, we were told that the figure was about 25 percent. Later, we understood how this figure was calculated. If one takes into account all the things that can go wrong, the final figure that emerges is about 5 percent.

Peter: What is meant here is that cell division and implantation is successful in about 25 percent of cases. After all, if all goes well up to that point, this can be counted as success, too.

Inge: But if you take it up to the real thing (a live baby at the end), the rate is only 5 percent. When I first heard 25 percent I thought, "That's not bad, I'll try it, perhaps we'll be lucky."

Peter: At that particular time there was a general euphoria in Germany. The first test-tube baby had been born in the Federal Republic only a few months before and Inge was immediately accepted because she was young and healthy.

Inge: We thought that it did not entail much surgery. I did not want to have a full-scale operation. The laparoscopy was a bad enough shock for my system. I am no hero when it comes to surgery, and a full anesthetic takes a lot out of me. When we heard that no major operation was involved, we thought that we could risk it.

Later, we also had moral scruples. For instance, when T told me that there were two egg cells and only one was to be put back as the other had not divided, I began to agonize over the thought that T might have not told me the truth: had he really collected more than one egg cell? And had he perhaps put them all back? How come only one had divided? What about the other(s)? I had this horror vision that somewhere a test-tube was bubbling over with a baby of mine! I know this is a mad idea, but I just cannot help imagining it; it has become an obsession: a baby appears, is suddenly there all alone in the test-tube...terrible, I could not sleep while I was thinking about it. Then it dies. Of course, what else can it do in a test-tube? Nothing happens with it, so it dies.

Peter: I must say, we were quite worried about how little support the women received. For instance, when they had to wait with a full bladder for their ultrasound test.

Inge: Fortunately, I was never alone, my sister was with me. But those others! When they talked about their lives, the hopes they invested, and the way they were treated! They tried to do everything right, to please T and his assistants. They were totally at their mercy. Disgusting! I thought, no, I am not going to be like that. I won't let them do that to me. I never had the slightest confidence in T. I did not know him, and he never behaved in a way that could have won my confidence. So why should I have believed him?

We tried IVF in September, and in the following spring we read about the controversy in England about how long embryos can be kept alive for research. The very thought made me sick! That is the reason why it is so important to trust the doctor and see a gynecologist whom one knows. I must be convinced that he does the job as an alternative for me and not for research.

Ute: After what you've experienced, would you advise other women against IVF?

Inge: I could not say to a woman that she should not try it. I can understand why she would want to go for it. So I would say to her: "O.K., it will be nasty and you will suffer." But I would not say that she should not be allowed to try.

Ute: Do you sometimes think that you would like to have another try for yourself?

Inge: Not for myself. For myself I would never do it again. Only if Peter insisted would I do it. But I don't think he would. I think of all the things that can go wrong, and the direction into which they are moving. And with every woman who volunteers, the doctors have won something. It helps them to improve their routine. No, I would not like to be part of their machinery ever again.

When You Must be in the Hospital

Most people are apprehensive about going to the hospital. Whether for surgery or for illness, a hospital stay is seldom number one on anyone's "things-I'd-love-to-do" list.

For most infertile couples, a stay at the hospital implies seeking a solution for their infertility, either through an operation for endometriosis (without hysterectomy) or for an in vitro fertilization/embryo transfer.

Medicine today sets its own priorities and terms. Physicians control about 70 percent of medical decision-making as well as the resource allocation process. The medical industry decides what will be taught in medical schools, how it will be taught, and what medical services will be offered, when, and where. Lack of foresight is a major problem in medical care today. For example, 95 percent of doctors now specialize in some form or other of medicine, even though it is predicted that by 1990 there will be a shortage of some 16,000 primary care physicians (general practitioners).

Because of the medical industry's monopoly on health care, more than twenty million Americans have inadequate access to quality medical care, and insurance costs are skyrocketing. There is also a rise in corporations that specialize in medical care— profit-making chains that operate "emergency rooms," laboratories and, now, mobile CAT scanners.

Much tax money is involved in public utilities and public education, and we expect some accountability from these industries; the medical industry, however, remains unaccountable to the public despite the fact that research, medical education, and hospitals are heavily subsidized by the taxpayer.

For most of us, the problems of hospitalization are cost, risk, isolation and, in almost all instances, the lack of accountability on the part of the physician and the hospital. We need to learn how to use hospitals because, chances are, most of us will have to use them at one time or another.

Before Entering the Hospital

Once the need for surgery has been confirmed with her doctor, a woman needs to know if the procedure to be accomplished is necessary or elective (not an emergency). Then, a second or even a third opinion should be sought.

She needs to know if there is more than one hospital in the community (sometimes, in small towns, people have little choice as one hospital serves several communities).

After the second/third opinion confirms the first opinion, the patient should again visit her doctor with a list of questions. She would be wise to schedule the appointment far enough in advance to give her time to think about her concerns and write them down. It is easier to discuss the surgery and what can be expected afterward when facing the doctor across his/her desk rather than lying naked and tranquilized on a medical table with feet in stirrups and posterior exposed.

Discuss finances. Some physicians settle for what the insurance company pays for a particular procedure; however, other physicians want their full fee, and the patient is responsible for the difference. Some doctors even require a down payment of 10 to 20 percent, particularly if s/he has had problems with the patient's carrier, or if the patient is insured by only one company. One should not be reticent about asking the physician about finances. Anyone about to enter a hospital has the right to know about financial matters ahead of time and not be surprised, perhaps unpleasantly, later.

Before entering the hospital, the patient would be wise to check with her insurance carrier to see what her policy covers and what it does not cover. Here again, the patient may be in for a surprise. Some companies, for example, that may not cover doctor's visits may cover the cost of seeking a second opinion. Other companies set limits on what they will pay to the doctor, anesthesiologist, assisting physician, etc. Policies come in all sizes, shapes, and scopes, and it is far better to be safe than sorry.

If a woman is employed, she will want to find out what kind of insurance her employer has. Some employers pay full salary for the entire length of incapacity; others have neither insurance nor disability pay. Sometimes, one can negotiate with the employer by using a combination of accrued sick and vacation time for the hospital stay and recuperation period.

If possible, the patient should choose the hospital where she will stay. Most doctors, except those in very small towns, have privileges in more than one hospital; therefore, if a woman has a preference, she should make her wishes known. She might consider which hospital is closer to her home, has the fewest traffic and parking problems (so family and friends can visit easily), and presents an environment she finds comfortable.

Check out the hospital with friends who have been there. Does the hospital consider special diet problems? Offer vegetarian meals? Have private rooms? Low-cholesterol meals? Whatever the patient's particular need may be, she needs to check to see if the hospital of her choice can fulfill those needs.

Before entering the hospital, contact the hospital's patient representative. Although this individual is usually employed by the hospital, s/he serves as a patient advocate. In addition to handling pre-admission problems, the patient representative helps patients with a wide variety of concerns, including questions about the patient's treatment.

If the hospital of choice does not have a patient representative, the patient might want to consider having her surgery at a hospital that does provide this service.

Anyone planning to enter a hospital for surgery or other procedure would be wise to practice good health habits prior to surgery so that recovery is quick and uneventful. Eat a high protein diet and maintain good digestion with high fiber foods. Supplements should include the vitamin B complex and vitamin C, both involved in healing and assisting the body to cope with stress. Skip processed foods, sugars, fats, and refined foods. If overweight, try to lose a few pounds.

With the coming of AIDS, a surgery patient ought to consider donating several units of her own blood in advance of the surgery, just in case it is needed.

There is evidence that tobacco smoke damages the body's ability to tolerate anesthesia and may cause short or long term complications. If the patient smokes, she may wish to quit for awhile before surgery.

The patient probably will have to visit the hospital a few days prior to scheduled surgery for blood tests, an electrocardiogram, chest X-ray, and urine tests. Some physicians also schedule an ultrasound test prior to the patient's entering the hospital.

Before entering the hospital, the patient needs to check if there are any rules about what clothing she should bring. Because of the possibility of theft, it is wise to leave valuables at home. The patient should check on visiting hours and advise her family to adhere to them, unless she wishes to make other arrangements with the hospital.

In the Hospital

Almost before the patient has a chance to take her shoes off, she usually will be asked to sign one or more consent forms. Her doctor will explain these and give her enough time to read them. If she is not happy with the form(s), she should immediately check the offending section(s) with the doctor or her patient representative. If it is something she feels strongly about, she might even want to consider calling her attorney. It has been suggested that these forms be signed several days prior to admission, but some hospitals do not allow this.

If the patient prefers to be alone, she can request that no visitors be allowed; however, it is a good idea to let someone close drop by because, often, that person is in a better position than the patient to see if all is as it should be and perhaps intervene if it is not.

Family and friends can be "watchdogs" for the patient because they are in a position to inquire about "oddities" in food or medication. Mistakes do occur—it's much better to avoid them.

The patient will be asked if she wants telephone service, television, or newspaper delivery. Today, most hospitals have television sets in each room. For the first two or three days after surgery, most patients are too uncomfortable or too "out of it" to care about any diversions, but later these can be helpful in the recovery process.

When there is abdominal surgery, expect to have the pubic hair shaved, an enema given, and to be taken off solid food for a minimum of twelve hours prior to surgery.

Whenever anyone is in the hospital, s/he has the right to know the name of one doctor in charge of her/his case. Whenever tests or X-rays are proposed, find out why. Remember that the rapid expansion of technology in hospitals not only greatly increases costs, but it also further depersonalizes care; therefore, such technology is often applied inappropriately and can cause iatrogenic (doctor caused) illnesses and other problems.

Smart patients make friends with the nursing staff. Nurses are the ones who coordinate patient care, and they keep their own records separately from the doctors'. Nurses' judgments can influence the entire course of the patient's care; however, they work under constraints that may limit their ability to advocate for the patient.

Try to go home as soon as possible. Not only are many hospitals crowded, but most suffer continuous outbreaks of infection that are becoming increasingly resistant to antibiotics. Called nosocomial infections, they are not brought in from outside the hospital but are produced within the hospital environment, mostly by the careless antiseptic practices of physicians and nurses.

In some operations, local anesthesia can be used rather than a general anesthesia. A "local" allows much quicker recovery and doesn't carry the same risk of death. The patient should urge her physician to use local anesthesia if at all possible.

Ask what medications have been prescribed, by whom, how often, and for what purpose. Ask the nurses what medication they are giving, and then check with the doctor. If possible, try not to take routine tranquilizers and sleeping pills. Instead of juice or any permitted "soft" drink, ask for milk at bedtime (it contains L-tryptophan, a natural relaxant), and this will probably eliminate the need for sleeping pills.

It has been shown repeatedly that hospital water at the patient's bedside is contaminated by bacteria, so consider bringing bottled water. Hospital food frequently is not nutritious, so ask friends to bring in some tasty, nourishing food. Unless the patient's doctor has a valid reason to object, take vitamins, particularly vitamin C.

Going Home

Before leaving the hospital, the patient needs to ask for a copy of her records. The hospital will probably send them to the patient's home. These records may prove useful in the future, particularly since some hospitals make it a policy to destroy records after a short time.

Recuperation time varies from three to eight weeks. Make sure to ask the doctor how long it will take before regular activities can be resumed safely. Hopefully, the patient planned ahead for people to help her with meals and to visit during those first few weeks at home.

Sometimes, when recuperation appears slow, depression and boredom set in. The patient might want to create a "recovery project" for those weeks at home. Sometimes, women confront "unfinished business" after surgery. They find this is an ideal time to face life issues that have been repressed and that suddenly come to light. If there is depression and confusion after surgery, the patient might want to consider finding a well-recommended professional counselor to help her sort out her feelings.

Try to relax. Recuperation seems so slow, but if the patient thinks of this time as an opportunity to learn and to grow, as a period of introspection and retrospection, she will find the time passing more quickly. If her surgery was an in vitro fertilization and embryo transfer, and she has conceived, she may soon embark on the most dangerous and exciting adventure in her life—motherhood.

A Hospital Patient's Bill of Rights

The following statement of patients' rights was prepared by the American Hospital Association's Committee on Health Care and distributed to member hospitals in the United States.

The patient has a right to:

1. Considerate and respectful care.
2. Obtain from her or his physician complete current information concerning diagnosis, treatment, and prognosis in terms the patient can reasonably be expected to understand.
3. Receive from her or his physician information necessary to give informed consent prior to the start of any procedure and/or treatment.
4. Refuse treatment to the extent permitted by law, and to be informed of the medical consequences of his or her action.
5. Every consideration of his or her privacy concerning his or her own medical program.
6. Expect that, within its capacity, a hospital must make reasonable response to the request of a patient for its services.
7. Expect that all communications and records pertaining to his or her care be treated as confidential.
8. Obtain information as to any relationship of her or his hospital to other health care and educational institutions insofar as her or his care is concerned.
9. Be advised if the hospital proposes to engage in or perform human experimentation affecting his or her care or treatment.
10. Expect reasonable continuity of care.
11. Examine and receive an explanation of her or his bill regardless of source of payment.
12. Know what hospital rules and regulations apply to his or her conduct as a patient.

SECTION 7

Learning Through Personal Experiences

Anne

When I was thirty-seven, I married a most compatible man and decided that we must have a child together, although I already had a six-year-old son by my first husband. I threw away my Pill packets and happily began looking for baby clothes. This second marriage was so full of love and optimism, in contrast to my first, that I wanted to express my happiness by creating a child. Six months passed and nothing happened, so I consulted my gynecologist, who started me on Clomid. I was already charting my basal body temperature along with my periods, trying to make love at the right time. Since a number of my friends had taken Clomid to ensure ovulation, I thought it was a good idea. I was not in the habit of questioning doctors, thinking they knew what they were doing. This man had a good reputation, so Jim and I said we'd go for it.

However, Clomid made me terribly nervous and anxious, and my peace of mind was shattered. On days off—you begin the drug on the third day of your cycle and take it for five days—I tried to regain my emotional balance and keep track of when to have intercourse. I can't say this helped our love life, but we were rewarded with a pregnancy.

At six weeks, however, I miscarried. It was a tremendous letdown for both of us because, by this time, Jim was as involved in making a baby as I was. He'd never been a father and, at age forty-five, regarded a pregnancy not only as a symbol of our love but as a sign of his vigor. Because of these feelings, we didn't hesitate to try again, and I went on Clomid, trying to accept the terrible feelings it caused in me. The doctor emphasized that time was against us if we didn't try again fast.

When I miscarried the second time, I was much more dejected and less enthusiastic about continuing this medical treatment. My physician had scheduled me to begin another round of Clomid the upcoming Monday, but a friend referred me to a health counselor with an interest in my problem. This woman took a careful history, asking me about the shape of my life—

relations with my child as well as with my husband, what we ate, and what amount of alcohol we used on a regular basis.

Since I have dieted for my entire life—I wear a size eight and have done some modeling—my report was not promising. I was embarrassed to tell the counselor that my mother had put me on a diet at age nine; my friends were all on diets of one kind or another and, currently, I took over-the-counter diet pills every day, not seeing any connection between them and my alleged infertility.

I changed these harmful eating patterns which, it appears, are not the best to conceive a child. Since my periods had not always been irregular before going on the Pill, and more recently on Clomid, I had a fair chance of regulating my own periods by improving health all around. Jim, an avid physical fitness enthusiast, liked this approach, although we understood that time was indeed a factor. However, the counselor explained that declining fertility as it related to my age had never been studied in terms of nutritional well-being. After all, up to 70 percent of all women in their late thirties can become pregnant within one year. Others might become pregnant by waiting longer or, like me, trying to improve general health.

In our meetings with this counselor—who, by the way, charged a fraction of a doctor's visit—we began to realize that we'd put happiness on hold and made infertility the focus of our lives. This attitude changed the relationship with my son, with Jim, and with my friends, whom I had dropped because I was so busy going to the doctor. Motivation is high when you're trying to get pregnant, so I tossed out the diet drugs and began to eat real food on a regular basis. We both took raw wheat germ, wheat germ oil, and 600 units of vitamin E daily. We concentrated on preparing lots of whole grain foods and fresh, organic vegetables.

After one month, the first change I noticed was energy; I stopped being tired. I found I could handle my strong-willed son again with patience and understanding. When I'd been overly preoccupied with my infertility, I was too busy with my new love and trying to make a baby. Now, I was present again for the child who was already with us, and he responded positively to this attention, making life easier for us all.

It took two years for me to become pregnant and, yes, we are very pleased about it, but this testimony does not end my story. I also want to call attention to pressures that push women like me to crazy diets and diet pills. For too long, my appearance defined my identity, and it will take more than a baby to change all of this negative programming. My problem, you see, was not infertility, but hatred for my own body—unless it stayed unreasonably thin. I'm sure other "infertile" women might want to know about this.

By *Margot Edwards; R.N., M.A.*

Story by an Older Mom

When we left the delivery room with our first child, my husband and I looked back to a problem-free pregnancy and a picture book delivery, despite the fact that my gynecological history had not been entirely uneventful.

Eighteen months later, I was wheeled into the emergency room with a ruptured ovarian cyst. Recovery was extremely slow, and I did not feel healthy for months. Just as my daughter was going through the terrible twos, my job became more stressful. We decided to take a leave and go abroad for six months on a project. I started a running program that I enjoyed tremendously. We then decided to have another baby and, after our first experience, we felt this would be easy.

A year went by and nothing happened. I tried to get my mind off the subject, and so I trained for a marathon. A week before the big race, I found myself in the emergency room again, this time for an ectopic pregnancy. My recovery was swift—after all, I was trained to run twenty-six miles.

The sadness persisted, but I kept running and finally gave up the last few cigarettes I still smoked. We always had an extremely healthy diet, including lots of whole grains, fresh fruits, and vegetables. I had given up coffee some time ago.

Ten months later, I had a positive pregnancy test, and we were elated. This time, things would work out (a serum pregnancy test had ruled out an ectopic pregnancy). I didn't mind my twenty-four-hour "morning" sickness and looked forward to another problem-free pregnancy.

Twelve weeks later, I started spotting and, when no heartbeat was detected, I had to face reality once more: suction curettage. Another life, another dream had ended all too soon. Again, my physical recovery was swift, but I was crushed. I could not, would not, did not accept that it happened to us again. I knew I could not disregard it this time and began to see a counselor. I also had a massage regularly—it was time to pamper myself.

Running, a good diet, and vitamin supplementation were not quite enough. I began to experiment with herbs, had a fertility mix prepared, and discovered that I had not forgotten the once- acquired technique of progressive relaxation. Two months later, I felt that, somehow, I was more balanced, more at peace with myself.

We moved to Switzerland, where I sought a good herb store and connected to other homeopathy-oriented people. Six months later, I was pregnant again and frightened. How could something we longed for so much be so scary? In the very conservative medical environment we were in, it was difficult to find the right doctor. I knew I would be treated as a high-risk patient with all of the latest technology forced on me. I compromised and settled for a doctor I knew was competent, but in so doing, I also knew that I would have to fight at times.

At ten weeks, an ultrasound revealed a live and thriving fetus. I had a new herbal pregnancy tea mix prepared. Walking had replaced running, and I walked at least three miles a day. We decided to have an amniocentesis this time, and we were overjoyed that everything was fine; however, even at twenty weeks, I could not quite embrace the pregnancy fully. Only at thirty weeks did I lose my fears, and I thoroughly enjoyed the last trimester.

I made another trip to the herbalist and had a birthing tea and a nursing mix prepared. My work load lightened as the academic year wound down, and I grew heavier. My due date came and went without any sign of the baby. For three weeks, the doctor told me that I was beginning to dilate and labor could start at any time.

One day after the due date, he called me into the hospital for monitoring. Everything was fine, but I knew the pressure was on. He was about to go on vacation and wanted to induce labor in three days. I was torn. I knew I did not want to jeopardize this pregnancy, but I also knew that induced labor was much harder, with one intervention often leading to the next.

In total despair, I called up my midwife, who was to come and check on me and the baby after we returned from the hospital (I registered for an ambulatory delivery that allowed the baby and me to go home a few hours after delivery). The midwife supported my decision to wait for another week—provided the baby was fine—and told me to inform the doctor the next morning.

To relax that evening, I prepared some birthing tea, had my husband give me a massage, and hoped that the full moon would do the rest. During the early morning hours, I went into labor. We went to the hospital when my contractions were about five minutes apart and my waters were leaking. The same midwife who had done the monitoring three days earlier welcomed us again. After the usual preparations, the fetal monitor was installed for twenty minutes. Everything was fine: I was at three centimeters. It took an hour to advance another centimeter, and the doctor indicated that, if I didn't progress faster, he would stimulate labor. We later learned that there were six women in labor, and the births were to be staggered according to the hospital's needs. I was furious!

My patience with authoritarian medicine ran out. I got up and announced in an authoritative voice that my husband and I were going for a walk and wanted to know when we had to be back. We were given an hour. During that hour, we walked briskly, did exercises to stimulate labor, and vowed to follow through with our own birth plan.

Forty minutes later, we barely made it back to the labor room, and I was at seven centimeters. Once again, the fetal monitor was installed—protest was futile—and removed as soon as I was moved to the delivery room.

It took only a few pushes before our healthy baby boy was born. We were elated and glad to leave the regimentation of the hospital a few hours later. In a country where women still stay in the hospital for four to seven days after childbirth, this was unusual. The nurses in the nursery loaded hot water bottles and glucose water on us, afraid the baby would not make it through the night without their supervision. I could not tell them that all he needed for his nutrition was colostrum and, to stabilize his temperature, he would sleep on my chest that night. They could not, would not, have understood that there is no need to intervene; nature provides all that is necessary.

Six weeks post-partum, I returned to running, equipped with a good sports bra made specifically for nursing mothers. Kevin Patrick is thriving, and my husband and I often wonder how we could have had such a perfect pregnancy and easy birth after so much trouble.

We were more inclined, perhaps, to compromise after losing two pregnancies, but we knew ourselves well enough to reject technological intervention when no particular need was convincingly established. I am happy that I will never know what might have happened had the doctor gotten his way and induced labor. We trusted in nature; the doctor, somehow, had lost that trust.

Some Helpful Herbs

For Fertility Mix:	Red Clover	
	Nettle Leaves	
	Red Raspberry	
	Dong Quai	MultiVitamin Complex
	False Unicorn	Extra B Complex
	Damiana	Royal Jelly (400 Mg. per day)
During Pregnancy Mix:	Red Raspberry	
	Alfalfa	
	Comfrey	
	Borage	
	Mint	Ultra Pre-Natal Complex
	Nettle	Extra B Complex
	Clover	Royal Jelly (200 Mg. per day)
Birthing Tea Mix:	Basil	
	Lavender	
	Nutmeg	
	Red Raspberry	
Breastfeeding Mix:	Fennel	
	Spearmint	
	Anise	
	Chamomile	
	Blessed Thistle	
	Borage	
	Bayberry	
	Milkwort	
	Hops	
	Lemon Grass	
	Red Raspberry	

By *Barbara Mercer*

Peter Pan Meets Miranda

As a couple, Jeff and I seem to have our most vital discussions when we are doing our most everyday chores. So it was that we were chopping vegetables for our Christmas Eve salad when we decided to see a doctor about why we weren't getting pregnant. After nearly two years of trying, it seemed like it was time. Nature just wasn't taking her course.

Our decision to have a child had not come easily—or even simultaneously. Being of the generation that pushed back childbearing from the age of twenty to thirty, we lacked the impetus of the traditional cultural norm to hurl us into precipitous parenthood. In fact, in the early years of our relationship we never even discussed kids.

When the subject finally did come up, we found we were of completely different minds. I first became aware of wanting to be a mother through a series of invisible experiences. In my mind's eye, I saw a curly-headed toddler running through the house; the chatter in my mind came to include the sounds of a baby's cry; and strange twinges came over my body when I saw a pregnant woman. When I heard myself tell a friend that my dozens of avocado plants were my babies, I realized what was really going on inside—that I had more emotional energy than I knew what to do with.

Jeff's experience was very different. In short, he had no interest in kids—a feeling that he put forth in two basic arguments: he was too young, and he didn't want to leave the work of the world to the next generation. He summed up his feelings in a simple phrase—he said he was suffering from the Peter Pan syndrome.

We spent a lot of time discussing whether to have or not to have; more often, we abandoned discussions entirely and fought. At the same time, we were somewhat appalled to find ourselves locked in this classic male/female struggle. We prided ourselves on being beyond the stereotypes, yet here we were, playing out of social conditioning.

Eventually, dogged persistence triumphed over confused resistance.

Reluctantly, Jeff agreed to give it a try, buoyed by the knowledge that two other couples whom we worked with were also packing in their diaphragms in favor of the next generation.

Having travailed through the really difficult task of decision making, I expected to get pregnant immediately. After all, we were in excellent health. Just as the commercial said, we ate right and got plenty of exercise. Even more to the point was the fact that my menstrual cycle had always been regular, tuned to the clock of the full moon. Besides all that, we had learned in junior high that nothing was easier than making babies.

And so it appeared, watching the parade of progeny passing before our lives. The experiences of our friends read like a verse from Genesis. Jan and Eddie gave birth to Micah; Joan and Tom bore Jeremy. Johanna was born to Andy and Bob; two Kates were born as second daughters. Neighbors, friends, and relatives—all were having children; people who were married, and those who were not. People who planned to have children and those who did not. Everyone was having babies—everyone but us.

The possibility of not being able to conceive had never occurred to us. Soon this thought came to dominate us. We looked for information. I read books on fertility and became versed in the vagaries of ovulation. I studied up on lunaception and learned how to chart my daily temperature.

When I went for my annual gynecological checkup, I took along my carefully plotted charts. The doctor studied them, pointed to a particular spot on the curve, and told me she thought I was pregnant. She also covered her bases by telling me to keep up the good work and come back with six months' more of charts, just in case she was wrong.

She was. It wasn't long before I wanted to throw the thermometer against the wall rather than put it in my mouth one more time. I came to hate graph paper and bristled when I saw numbers like ninety-seven and ninety-eight. The daily monitoring of my vital signs, coupled with the well-intentioned but thoroughly useless advice of friends not to try so hard, began to drive me crazy.

I threw away the charts but couldn't escape the private thought that something was wrong with us. Yet, we couldn't quite believe that biology was the only force at work. It was impossible to ignore Jeff's case of chronic ambivalence. Perhaps he had stumbled upon the world's solution to birth control. If only he could bottle it and find the appropriate distribution mechanism, he might become the Margaret Sanger of the late twentieth century.

Eventually, we started talking with other people about what was happening or, to be more precise, what was not happening. It was a relief to learn that we were not the only couple to have had this experience. We heard of couples who had tried for as many as seven years—then, without explanation, conceived. Three-, four-, and five-year-long attempts were not uncommon, even among couples who had gone through the medical checkout and been given a discouraging prognosis. A new truth began to emerge—the great hush-hush secret of our time—getting pregnant was not always all that easy.

All this information helped, but it was hardly a substitute for a baby. I found various ways to surround myself with baby energy. I borrowed a crib from a friend whose kids were grown. I volunteered to work in the day care cooperative that had been formed for Micah, Jeremy, and Johanna. I sat with my friends while they nursed their babies. In my own way, I created a private, ongoing fertility rite.

In spite of creating my own mythology, and Jeff's evolving desire to become a father, the months just ticked on by. Every few months or so, I thought I was pregnant. I was always wrong.

Such was our situation as we tossed our Christmas Eve salad and discussed our options. I was feeling my all-too-familiar premenstrual symptoms when we agreed to see a doctor after the first of the year and talked, for the first time, about adoption.

One week went by, then another. Something was very strange. My period never came. Afraid to believe what, in retrospect, seems so very obvious for fear of disappointment, we only alluded to the possibility obliquely to each other. Finally, we were willing to risk resolving the ambiguity and carried a small specimen to a nearby medical lab. Seven hours later, the voice of a complete stranger brought me the news that I was pregnant.

It was a telephone call which marked the beginning of a transformative experience for both of us. I relished every moment of the pregnancy and reveled in every pound I gained. I loved every little twitch and kick the baby made. I dreamt about having quintuplets. The due date came and went as due dates tend to do. Having waited so long to conceive, we could hardly expect the baby to be early. We considered naming her Patience.

As for Jeff—the man who never wanted children—he followed every step of the pregnancy, taking pictures and talking about the changes that awaited us. When our doctor suggested that Jeff be the one to "catch the baby," he rose to the occasion. He eased Miranda from the womb, placed her on my stomach, cut her umbilical cord, and gave her the Leboyer bath. Some hours after the birth, he started to cry, overcome by the wonder of it all, saying over and over that he couldn't believe how instantly and how much he loved her. I wonder what Peter Pan would think of that?

By *Jessica Lipnack*

A Word on Waiting

It took my husband and me three long years to conceive our first child. The period in our lives that sometimes seemed like an endless trial has had a happy ending and a new beginning. Our daughter, Flora Jane, is now twenty months old. The sadness that once filled my heart at the thought of never being fortunate enough to bear a child has vanished, replaced by the fresh morning breeze of our little girl.

A while ago, when I was expounding in a rather lofty fashion to a pregnant friend about all the insight and wisdom her childbirth labor would bring her, her husband turned to me and said, "Pretty easy to be objective when you're six months down the road." Who am I to tell those of you who have waited long so to have a little baby of your own to relax? Yet, I've been there and back in all its flaming intensity and, honestly, that isn't the best way to go.

Probably many of you, like me, started popping birth control pills when you were too young to know any better and kept it up for a few years until your body yelled "STOP!" so loud you couldn't ignore it any longer. Then, in went the IUD while you pursued "you" and all those interests you were led to believe were so important—college, friends, travel. (A woman friend who knew her calling early on in life was told by her high school guidance counselor that he would not accept mothering as a career choice.) If a little voice inside said, "Wait a minute," you might have been moving too fast to hear. I know I was. I wanted to try this, that, and the other thing before settling down. I felt pity for the women I knew who were tied down before their time with little ones. I wasn't going to let that happen to me. No, sir. I was in control of my life.

Then comes the moment of decision when you finally decide, "This is it!" You catch yourself peeking in baby carriages and cuddling those sweet bundles close. A few of your friends have children and are doing well. I was lucky enough to have a close friend who loved mothering so much she glowed. She hugged me tight when I told her we decided to have a baby. She kept on hugging me tighter and tighter for the next three years as the roller coaster ride got scarier and crazier. Most of the time, I kept up a good front, but with this special woman, I just let go and held on.

It hurt a lot. Our initial anticipation and excitement gave way to sadness, emptiness, and finally courage. You need courage to try to accept the hand fate has dealt you and get on with your life. Melodramatic as this may sound, empty arms that long for a baby ache. Recently, at a La Leche League meeting where the mothers were talking about the experience of infant death, I became overwhelmed with grief and sorrow. I felt like crying my eyes out. Later, reflecting on my strong emotional reaction to this discussion, I realized my sense of loss over not being able to become pregnant was similar to that of a woman who experiences miscarriage or a stillbirth. The baby I longed for was real to me.

I don't want to dwell on the medical procedures we underwent to determine our physical ability to become pregnant, mainly because I do not place much faith in them anymore. We had a sperm count, a post-coital, and a hysterosalpingogram, in that order. If you feel inclined to check out the usual tests, it might set your mind at ease to know there's nothing wrong. For me, this knowledge did not balance out the humiliation and lack of compassion I felt after baring my soul in such an impersonal situation. Although we kept accurate records for many months of my cycle to determine my fertile days, that didn't help either. At that point, I was almost maniacally intent on having a baby. Perhaps if I had gone about the natural methods of family planning in a more relaxed fashion, we would have had a positive result sooner. The basal thermometer charts showed regular ovulation. I guess I just had a lot to learn before becoming a mama.

I tended to be one of those people who didn't appreciate what I had. I believe now I needed the waiting period to understand the blessing of motherhood. People tell me this isn't so. They say I'd have loved my children just as much whenever they'd come along. However, I was the only woman in my birth class who didn't have an ache or pain.

We'd pretty much given up when a teacher told us about an M.D.-chiropractor who was a spiritual healer. He was a man in his seventies, who spluttered into his walrus moustache when I mentioned a medical finding on infertility.

"Who told you that?" he boomed.

"Science," I answered meekly.

"HOGWASH!" he thundered, closing the discussion on science with a bang of his fist. After three treatments and a lot of parsley, I conceived.

Whether it was our doctor or not, who can say? I am thankful for his help. It was (finally) our time to have a child. I floated through the next nine months, forty-five pounds heavier in flesh but two tons lighter in spirit.

So many times, I hear women making plans to conceive a child in a month. I'm silent, allowing that we must all work out our lives in our own ways, but inside I'm saying, "Is that what really matters?" Were we really meant to plan out each trivial detail for the convenience of our own sense of order? Just because you feel it's the right time to have a baby doesn't necessarily mean it's the right time in the universe for that soul to be born. When someone asks me now if we plan to have more children or a large family, I answer, "We'll wait and see."

Statistics tell us that, today, one in five couples are infertile. What does that mean? Perhaps it means that, after not becoming pregnant at the planned time, the confused couple runs helter-skelter to the nearest specialist for help. Trying to become pregnant in the first place may be a mistake. When conception is not immediate, further attempts to solve the problem may cause more anxiety until you are nearly frantic. This state of emotional upheaval is not a good climate for a vessel to receive a new soul, and so, the soul may wait until you are calm and ready to receive it. Although I recognize that some infertility problems respond to medical treatment, I also wonder how many of these problems we create for ourselves.

If you are a woman who longs for a child and feels time passing away like a lead stone without one, take heart. Breathe deep. Feel peace. Meditate on mothering. Know that your mothering spirit wishes to care for all, not just your own. Spread the love you want to shower on your children to others—your mate, your parents, your friends. Share your goodness with those around you, both young and old. If there is a knot of anxiety in your heart, as there was in mine, talk to someone close who will value your feelings. Listen to your heartsong. Eat nourishing food. Be thankful. Through this waiting period, you may gain more than you could ever believe possible.

By *Cheryl Downing*

GLOSSARY

Glossary

Acupuncture. Balancing treatment that increases vitality, reduces pain, and improves reproductive function. Fine needles applied at key points are relatively painless and quite relaxing. Used in conjunction with herbals for selected infertility problems.

Adhesions. Scar tissue that appears inside the body after infection, inflammation, or surgery. Adhesions block passage of egg or sperm and interfere with implantation.

AI. Artificial insemination is the process of depositing sperm near the cervix or directly into the uterus when there is a male infertility problem.

AID. Artificial insemination with donor sperm. Also referred to as DI (donor insemination).

AIH. Artificial insemination with husband's sperm.

Amenorrhea. Absence of menstruation, "primary" when the woman has never menstruated; "secondary" when a woman with a history of menstruation stops having periods for six months or longer. Secondary amenorrhea is normal during pregnancy and lactation and after the menopause.

Anovulation. Absence of ovulation.

Azoospermia. Absence of sperm in a semen sample due to sperm production problem and/or blocked vas deferens.

BBT. Basal body temperature, the resting body temperature taken upon awakening, has a "biphasic" pattern in the monthly cycle, shifting from a pre-ovulatory low to a post-ovulatory high (.5 degree rise) when ovulation occurs. An anovulatory cycle is "monophasic" or constant for the entire month.

Biofeedback. Relaxation training using technical "feed back" to reinforce learning. Usually, a hand-held or desktop device measures galvanic skin response, pulse rate, and brain waves to indicate whether or not a person is in the relaxed "alpha" brain wave state.

Bromocriptine. Parlodel, a drug used to reduce excess levels of prolactin for infertility and, after childbirth, to suppress lactation when a woman prefers bottle-feeding. Unwanted side effects include headache, dizziness, and nausea. Rare, but reported, are seizures.

Cervical mucus. Secretions of cervical glands that change consistency at various phases of the menstrual cycle. Infertile mucus is thick and inhospitable to sperm. Fertile mucus is thin and hospitable to sperm. A simple way to determine whether or not fertile mucus is present is to study the Fertility Awareness Method.

Cervix. The neck of the uterus that opens into the vagina. The cervix changes position and consistency under the influence of hormones during the monthly cycle. An "incompetent" or loose cervix can lead to miscarriage as pregnancy advances.

Clomiphene citrate. A drug marketed as Clomid or Serophene used to induce ovulation. It stimulates the pituitary to produce FSH and LH in larger quantities than usual in order to produce multiple eggs and increase the chances of a pregnancy. Unwanted side effects include hot flashes and PMS symptoms: nervousness, anxiety, and hostility.

Coitus. Medical terminology for sexual intercourse.

Corpus luteum. Yellow body that appears at the site where the egg was released from the follicle. Produces progesterone to support a pregnancy.

Danocrine. A male hormone marketed as Danazol that is prescribed for endometriosis to suppress ovulation and, hopefully, "dry up" endo implants so a woman can become pregnant. Side effects include weight gain and masculinizing effects.

DES. Diethylstilbestrol, an estrogen drug prescribed in the past to prevent miscarriage (ineffectual). Offspring (DES sons and daughters) were born with abnormalities of the reproductive organs that cause infertility problems. Some DES daughters suffered a rare form of vaginal cancer.

Dysmenorrhea. Painful menstrual periods.

Dyspareunia. Painful intercourse.

Ectopic pregnancy. A pregnancy that implants outside of the uterus, frequently in the fallopian tube. If rupture occurs, it constitutes a medical emergency. Ectopic pregnancy occurs at a higher rate in I.U.D.-users.

Egg retrieval. Surgically removing eggs from the ovary for in vitro fertilization or gamete intrafallopian transfer. Aspiration of the eggs is conducted through a laparoscope or with ultrasound guiding the needle through vagina, bladder, or abdomen (UDOR— ultrasonically directed oocyte retrieval or TUDOR—transvaginal UDOR).

Ejaculate. Semen made up of sperm and secretions from the seminal vesicles, prostate, and Cowper's glands.

Ejaculation. Expelling semen, usually during orgasm. Ejaculation does not occur with some male sexual dysfunctions.

Embryo. Fertilized egg as it develops during the first eight weeks of pregnancy.

Embryo transfer. If in vitro fertilization is successful, living embryos are transferred from a dish into a woman's uterus where, hopefully, one will implant.

Endometrial biopsy. Surgically removing a piece of the endometrium to determine whether or not ovulation has occurred.

Endometriosis. Tissue that ordinarily lines the inside of the uterus is located elsewhere. Under the influence of hormones, it bleeds monthly, causing inflammation, pain, and, in some cases, infertility (by interfering with ovulation and implantation).

Epididymis. Storage area for sperm where it matures before moving into vas deferens. Located above the testes.

Estrogen. An ovarian hormone that stimulates follicle development, endometrial growth, and the appearance of fertile mucus in the pre-ovulatory phase of the menstrual cycle. Estrogen is also responsible for the LH surge, a spike in the luteinizing hormone that triggers ovulation. In puberty, estrogen causes secondary sex characteristics to develop.

Fertile mucus patch. Period when fertile mucus can be detected.

Fertility Awareness Method. Systematic way to predict fertile days by tracking changes in cervical mucus, cervical position, and BBT. Not to be confused with the ineffectual Rhythm Method, Fertility Awareness is also a family planning method as effective as the Pill. Also known as the Ovulation Method, Sympto-Thermal Method, Mucus Method, and Billings Method (philosophies vary in each method, but all use the same evaluations).

Fertilization. Egg and sperm unite, usually in a fallopian tube.

Fetus. The baby in the uterus from eight weeks of pregnancy until birth.

Follicular phase. Pre-ovulatory phase of the menstrual cycle, also referred to as estrogen phase or proliferative phase.

FSH. Follicle stimulating hormone secreted by the brain to trigger sperm production in the testes or follicle development in the ovary.

GIFT. Gamete intrafallopian transfer, a surgical technique that aspirates eggs from the ovary and places them with the sperm directly into a fallopian tube where, hopefully, fertilization will occur. Used instead of in vitro fertilization in women with one functioning fallopian tube.

GnRH. Gonadotropin releasing hormone administered by nasal spray that triggers the pituitary gland to release FSH and LH. Used with induction of ovulation and as a treatment for endometriosis.

Hamster test. Sperm penetration test to evaluate whether or not sperm can penetrate a hamster egg.

HCG. Human chorionic gonadotropin, a hormone produced by the placenta in pregnancy, used as a fertility drug to trigger release of the egg.

HMG. Human menopausal gonadotropin marketed as Pergonal, a fertility drug used to induce ovulation. Pergonal contains a large concentration of FSH and LH that forces the ovary to work double time and produce multiple eggs. Two risks are hyperstimulation of the ovary and multiple births. Also involves daily injections and tests and is very expensive.

HSG. Hysterosalpingogram, an X-ray procedure that injects dye into the uterus to see whether or not it will spill out the fallopian tubes. Determines patency (if tubes are open). A safer water-based dye is used in China.

Hyperprolactinemia. Excess prolactin in the non-lactating woman that can suppress ovulation. Sometimes caused by stress.

Hysteroscopy. Examining the interior of the uterus with an instrument (hysteroscope) inserted through the cervix.

Hysterectomy. Removal of the uterus.

Hyperthyroidism. Overactive thyroid gland increases metabolism, which can destroy estrogen and thus interfere with ovulation.

Hypothyroidism. Underactive thyroid gland lowers metabolism which can increase prolactin levels in both sexes and cause women to produce too much estrogen.

ICSH. Interstitial cell stimulating hormone, the LH hormone in a male that triggers testes to produce sperm.

Immunological infertility. Male or female reaction against sperm.

Implantation. Fertilized egg implants into the lining of the uterus. The I.U.D. interferes with implantation.

IUI. Intrauterine insemination. Placing washed sperm directly into the uterus to increase the chances of fertilization. IUI/H uses husband's sperm; IUI/D uses donor sperm.

IVF. In vitro fertilization, a seven step process that fertilizes human eggs outside the body.

Karyotyping. Genetic test that analyzes chromosomes after repeated miscarriage or birth defect.

Laparoscopy. Visualizing abdominal organs through a telescope-like instrument in order to make a diagnosis and/or repair. Requires general anesthesia and two or three puncture wounds.

Laparotomy. Surgically opening the abdomen to make a diagnosis and/or repair. Major surgery.

LH. Luteinizing hormone secreted by pituitary gland triggers the testes to produce testosterone and the ovaries to produce progesterone.

LH surge. Spike in LH that precedes ovulation.

Lunaception. Process of manipulating light and darkness to regulate the menstrual cycle. Over-exposure to light during the night time hours can disrupt the menstrual cycle.

Luteal phase. Post-ovulatory phase of the menstrual cycle, also referred to as the progesterone phase or the secretory phase.

Luteal phase defect. Short post-ovulatory phase with insufficient production of progesterone.

Metrodin. Potent fertility drug used to induce superovulation.

Motility. Ability of sperm to swim in straight line.

Oligospermia. Low sperm count.

Oocyte. An immature egg.

Ovaries. Female gonads that produce estrogen, progesterone, and release one egg monthly.

Ovulation. Release of the egg at mid-cycle.

Ovulation induction. Artificially inducing ovulation with drugs.

Ovulation Method. Synonymous with Fertility Awareness Method and Mucus Method. Uses data taken from a woman's body (cervical mucus, position of cervix, BBT) to predict ovulation.

Ovulation predictors. Do-it-yourself urine tests (available at the drugstore) that signal the advent of ovulation before it occurs (urine changes color when LH surges). Marketed as First Response, OvuStick, and Cue.

Ovulation pump. Transportable pump used at home to administer GnRH.

PID. Pelvic inflammatory disease, infection of the reproductive organs, usually the fallopian tubes, caused most often by gonorrhea or chlamydia (which, in women, can be asymptomatic).

Pituitary gland. Master gland in the brain that produces FSH and LH to stimulate ovaries and testes. Part of a delicate relay system involved in reproduction, the pituitary is suppressed by the Pill.

Polycystic ovaries. Disease where ovaries produce cysts instead of releasing eggs.

Post-coital test. Test performed on cervical mucus two to three hours after intercourse to see how mucus and sperm interact. Evaluates whether or not sperm can swim through cervical mucus, if there is any clumping, and whether or not male or female antibodies to sperm are present.

Post Pill Syndrome. Failure to ovulate once a woman stops using the Pill, due to suppression of the pituitary gland.

Progesterone. An ovarian hormone that stimulates glandular development in the endometrium and elevates BBT in the post-ovulatory or luteal phase. Progesterone sustains a pregnancy.

Progesterone withdrawal. Used before inducing ovulation with fertility drugs to bring on the menstrual period.

Prolactin. A hormone produced by the pituitary gland that triggers lactation. When it's excessive in the non-lactating woman, it can suppress ovulation.

Self-help. Improving health with diet, biofeedback, and other low-tech interventions. Requires research and motivation.

Semen. Male ejaculatory fluid containing nourishing secretions from the Cowper's, seminal vesicles, and prostate glands to feed and protect sperm on its way to meet the egg.

Semen analysis. Basis of the male infertility workup. Evaluates semen volume, sperm shape and movement, sperm count, and any evidence of infection or antibodies to sperm.

Sperm antibodies. Antibodies in the male or female that attack sperm.

Sperm-mucus cross test. Microscopically determines whether or not antibodies are present by analyzing husband's sperm two ways: combined with his wife's cervical mucus; combined with bovine mucus. The wife's mucus mixed with donor sperm is also tested.

Split-ejaculate. Splitting semen sample to concentrate sperm for insemination. Most sperm is found in first portion of ejaculate.

TCM. Traditional Chinese medicine, an age-old system using acupuncture and herbs, among other treatments. Diagnosis relies upon a sophisticated system of pulse readings, among other assessments. TCM includes treatment for infertility, which can be quite effective in selected cases.

Testes. Male gonads that produce testosterone and manufacture sperm.

Testicular biopsy. Surgically removing a piece of the testes to determine whether or not it is normal.

Testosterone. A testicular hormone involved in producing sperm and maintaining libido (sexual desire) in male and female. (Note that men secrete small amounts of female sex hormones, just as women produce small amounts of male sex hormones.)

TUDOR. Transvaginal ultrasound directed oocyte retrieval, a surgical procedure using ultrasound instead of laparoscopy to aspirate eggs for in vitro fertilization or gamete intrafallopian transfer. Eliminates need for general anesthesia.

Ultrasound. Sound waves used instead of X-ray to visualize the body organs. Emits non-ionizing energy.

UDOR. Ultrasound directed oocyte retrieval, a surgical procedure using ultrasound instead of laparoscopy to aspirate eggs for in vitro fertilization or gamete intrafallopian transfer. Eliminates need for general anesthesia, using epidural, local, and sedation.

Varicocele. Enlarged vein in the testicle that is a major cause of male infertility.

Vas deferens. Passageway for sperm that runs from testes to urethra. In vasectomy, the vas deferens is cut to provide a permanent method of birth control.

Washed sperm. Processing the sperm to bring the best swimmers up to the top of a centrifuged sample. Used for insemination.

RECOMMENDED READINGS
and
ADDITIONAL RESOURCES

Recommended Readings

ACUPRESSURE FOR WOMEN by Cathryn Bauer, 1987, The Crossing Press, Freedom, CA.

ADOPTION; PARENTHOOD WITHOUT PREGNANCY by Charlene Canepe, 1986, Henry Hold & Co., NY.

THE ADOPTION RESOURCE BOOK by Ois Gilman, 1987, Harper & Row, NY.

BIRTH CONTROL AND CONTROLLING BIRTH: WOMAN-CENTERED PERSPECTIVES edited by Helen B. Holmes, Betty B. Hoskins, and Michael Gross, 1981, The Humana Press, Clifton, NY.

THE COMPLETE GUIDE TO WOMEN'S HEALTH by Bruce D. and Carroll A. Shephard, rev. 1988, New American Library, NY.

A COUPLE'S GUIDE TO FERTILITY: THE COMPLETE SYMPTO-THERMAL METHOD by R. J. Hunegar and Rose Fuller, 1986, Northwest NFP Services, 4805 NE Glison, Portland, OR 97213.

THE CUSTOM-MADE CHILD: WOMAN-CENTERED PERSPECTIVES edited by Helen B. Holmes, Betty B. Hoskins, and Michael Gross, 1981, The Humana Press, Clifton, NJ.

EMBRYOS, ETHICS AND WOMEN'S RIGHTS: EXPLORING THE NEW REPRODUCTIVE TECHNOLOGIES edited by Elaine Hoffman Baruch, Amadeo F. D'Amado, Jr., and Joni Seager, 1988, Harrington Park Press, NY.

THE EXPLOITATION OF A DESIRE: WOMEN'S EXPERIENCES WITH IN VITRO FERTILIZATION by Renate Klein, Women's Studies Summer Institute 1989, Deakin University Press, Deakin University, Geelong, Victoria, 3217, Australia.

A FERTILITY AWARENESS AND NATURAL FAMILY PLANNING RESOURCE DIRECTORY edited by Suzannah Cooper, 1988, Small World Publications, P.O. Box 305, Corvallis, OR 97339.

HAVING YOUR BABY BY DONOR INSEMINATION: A COMPLETE RESOURCE GUIDE by Elizabeth Noble, 1987, Houghton Mifflin, Boston.

"In Vitro Fertilization: Reflections on the State of the Art" by Helen B. Holmes, BIRTH: ISSUES IN PERINATAL CARE AND EDUCATION, September 1988.

INFERTILITY: A GUIDE FOR THE CHILDLESS COUPLE by Barbara Eck Menning, rev. 1988, Prentice-Hall, NY.

INFERTILITY AND BIRTH DEFECTS: IS MERCURY FROM SILVER DENTAL FILLINGS AN UNSUSPECTED CAUSE? by Sam Ziff and Dr. Michael F. Ziff, 1987, Bio-Probe, P.O. Box 580160, Orlando, FL 32858-0160.

THE INFERTILITY BOOK, A COMPREHENSIVE MEDICAL AND EMOTIONAL GUIDE by Carla Harkness, 1987, Volcano Press, San Francisco, CA.

INFERTILITY: HOW COUPLES CAN COPE by Linda P. Saltzer, 1986, G. K. Hall & Co., Boston.

THE INFERTILITY MAZE by Kassie Schwan, 1988, Contemporary Books, NY.

INFERTILITY TROUBLE-SHOOTING: SELF HELP SUGGESTIONS FOR REGAINING FERTILITY, by Suzannah Cooper, 1985, Small World Publications, P.O. Box 305, Corvallis, OR 97339.

INFERTILITY: WOMEN SPEAK OUT edited by Renate Klein, Pandora Press, London, Sydney.

MIRACLE BABIES AND OTHER HAPPY ENDINGS FOR COUPLES WITH FERTILITY PROBLEMS by Mark Perloe and Linda Gail Christie, 1987, Rawson Associates, NY.

THE MIRACLE SEEKERS: AN ANTHOLOGY OF INFERTILITY by Mary M. Mason, 1987, Prospect Pubs., Indiana.

THE MOTHER MACHINE: REPRODUCTIVE TECHNOLOGIES FROM ARTIFICIAL INSEMINATION TO ARTIFICIAL WOMBS by Gena Corea, 1986, Harper & Row, NY.

THE NEW OUR BODIES, OURSELVES by Boston Women's Health Book Collective, 1985, Simon & Schuster, NY.

NEW CONCEPTIONS: A CONSUMER'S GUIDE TO THE NEWEST INFERTILITY TREATMENTS by Lori B. Andrews, 1984, St. Martin's Press, NY.

OVERCOMING ENDOMETRIOSIS: NEW HELP FROM THE ENDOMETRIOSIS ASSOCIATION by Mary Lou Ballweg and the Endometriosis Association, 1987, Congdon & Weed, NY and Chicago.

THE PERSONAL FERTILITY GUIDE by Terrie Guay, rev. 1986, Beufort Books, NY.

RECREATING MOTHERHOOD: IDEOLOGY AND TECHNOLOGY IN A PATRIARCHAL SOCIETY by Barbara Katz Rothman, 1989, W. W. Norton, NY.

"The Risk of High Multiparity with IVF/ET" by Frances V. Price, BIRTH: ISSUES IN PERINATAL CARE AND EDUCATION, September 1988.

SIGNS OF FERTILITY: THE PERSONAL SCIENCE OF NATURAL BIRTH CONTROL by Margaret Nofziger Dotzler, 1988, MND Publishing, 7163 Old Harding Road, Nashville, TN 37221.

TEST-TUBE WOMEN: WHAT FUTURE FOR MOTHERHOOD edited by Rita Arditti, Renate Duelli Klein, and Shelly Minden, 1984, Pandora Press, Boston.

WISE WOMAN HERBAL by Susun B. Weed, 1985, Ash Tree Publishers, Woodstock, NY.

WITHOUT CHILD: EXPERIENCING AND RESOLVING INFERTILITY by Ellen Glazer and Susan Cooper, 1988, Lexington Books, D. C. Heath & Co., Lexington, MA and Toronto.

WOMANCARE, A GYNECOLOGICAL GUIDE TO YOUR BODY by Lynda Madaras and Jane Patterson, rev. 1984, Avon Books, NY.

WOMEN AND THE CRISIS IN SEX HORMONES by Barbara and Gideon Seaman, 1977, Rawson Associates, NY.

WOMEN'S HEALTH CARE: A GUIDE TO ALTERNATIVES edited by Kay Weiss, 1984, Reston Pub. Co.

Additional Resources

RESOLVE, Inc., 5 Water Street, Arlington, MA 02174 (617)643-2424
—a national nonprofit group offering information and support to infertile couples.

OVULATION METHOD TEACHERS ASSOCIATION (OMTA) P.O. Box 101780, Anchorage, AK 99510-1780 (907)343-4785
—national nonprofit group offering information, referral, and support for those wanting to know more about Fertility Awareness.

FERTILITY AWARENESS EDUCATION & SUPPORT Suzannah Cooper, Director, P.O. Box 305, Corvallis, OR 97339 (503)753-8530
—national resource and support group for teachers, researchers, the media, and the general public. Offers networking and consultation on Fertility Awareness.

AMERICAN FERTILITY SOCIETY 2131 Magnolia Avenue, Suite 201 Birmingham, AL 35256
—offers referral list of infertility physicians and counselors, and list of suggested reading on infertility. Publishes *Fertility* and*Sterility*.

FAMILY LIFE INFORMATION EXCHANGE (FLIE) Box 10716 Rockville, MD 20850 (301)770-3662
—national clearinghouse for family planning-related information. Offers free single copies of a bibliography listing infertility books and resources.

INDEX

Index